A new medical pluralism?
Alternative medicine, doctors, patients and the state

Sarah Cant and Ursula Sharma
Roehampton Institute London and
University of Derby

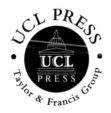

UCL PRESS
UCL
PRESS
Taylor & Francis Group

Published in the UK in 1999 by UCL Press

UCL Press Limited
Taylor & Francis Group
1 Gunpowder Square
London EC4A 3DF

Distributed in North America by

Garland Publishing
19 Union Square West
New York,
NY 10003-3382
USA

The name of University College London (UCL) is a registered trade
mark used by UCL Press with the consent of the owner.

ISBNs: 1-85728-510-7 HB
       1-85728-511-5 PB

British Cataloguing-in-Publication Data
A catalogue record for this book is available from the British Library.

Printed and bound by T.J. International Ltd, Padstow, Cornwall
Typeset by Best-set Typesetter Ltd., Hong Kong

A new medical pluralism?

For Elliot and Oliver,
born to Sarah during the making of this book.

CONTENTS

ACKNOWLEDGEMENTS

We have been conducting research on alternative medicines over a number of years, both severally and in collaboration. This book is the product of that work – we will not say "culmination" as we hope there is more to come! One very important phase of this programme of research, a project on "Professionalisation in complementary medicine", was funded by the ESRC whose support we gratefully recognize.

Many people have helped us in this work. We would particularly like to thank the publisher's anonymous referees whose comments we found most helpful. Our gratitude is also due to Louise Richards for helping to prepare the bibliography and Ulla Gustafsson for proof reading and comments.

Academics have a great deal to answer for to their families; we are truly appreciative of the support given by our partners and children. We hope that they feel that this book is a worthy tribute to their patience and practical help.

Most of all we would like to thank each other for mutual friendship, respect and inspiration.

CHAPTER 1

A new medical pluralism?

The re-emergence of complementary medicine in western countries

Pluralism in health care is nothing new. There has always been the possibility of choice between different kinds of practitioner, between consulting or self-prescribing, and there have always been multiple ways of understanding health and sickness. Yet in Britain, and in the West more generally, orthodox medicine has secured a position of social, economic and ideological hegemony in the health care market as a result of its own professional project and through the support of the state. This hegemonic position has been maintained for at least a century but since the late 1960s the growing popularity of "alternative" or "complementary" medicines might appear to be undermining it and bringing about a revival of pluralism.

In this book we attempt a sociological account of the florescence of these alternative medicines. While we shall focus primarily on Great Britain, we wish to set this material in a comparative framework, since what has been happening in Britain reflects much wider trends. The most relevant comparisons will be with other western European countries, North America and the other (mainly anglophone) countries that are generally referred to collectively as "the West" (a problematic term if ever there was one). Does the increased popularity of alternative medicines mean that we are witnessing a new form of medical pluralism? If so, what are its features and what kind of commentary upon it can we, as sociologists, provide? The issue of alternative medicine is neither trivial nor local. Many of the alternative healing therapies have professionalized rapidly in terms of training and organization, becoming much more vocal and confident. In the context of a widespread public health care funding crisis governments have slowly begun to take account of a possible role for alternative medicine in the overall health care system and some have begun to see its legitimation as a policy issue. National orthodox medical associations have felt called upon to take positions on the validity of complementary medicine and to consider its potential threat to their privileged positions. What has obliged both governments and doctors, more than anything else, to take these forms of healing very seriously has been the evidence of their enormous popular appeal.

Consultations with alternative practitioners account for a high proportion of total health care consultations, and private expenditure on such services is considerable. For example, a national study in the United States found that of a sample of 1,539 adults, 34 per cent had used at least one form of alternative therapy during the past year (Eisenberg et al. 1993). The authors of this study estimated that Americans made around 425 million visits to providers of unconventional medicine in the year 1990, more than the total number of visits to all US primary care physicians. A British study estimated that four million consultations took place in 1987, "roughly one for every 55 patient consultations with a general practitioner in the NHS" (Thomas et al. 1991). Surveys from other North European countries show similar statistics (e.g. Menges 1994), as do studies from Australia and New Zealand (e.g. MacLennan et al. 1996).

There is a paucity of such survey data from southern Europe (Spain, Portugal, Italy, Greece). Scattered research articles (e.g. Lalli 1983, Pereira 1993) and information from professional journals suggest that there is a significant degree of interest in alternative medicines in those areas. In the former Soviet bloc there appears to be an upsurge of interest in non-biomedical systems of healing (Suvorinova 1990) but at this moment it is difficult to gauge its volume and direction. Owing to the paucity of good quality and accessible research data we have not attempted to say very much about the former Soviet bloc in this book, an omission which we

2

hope to be able to remedy in the future. In eastern Europe there are many new training opportunities in modalities like homoeopathy, and in the countries of the former Soviet Union it is likely that various kinds of folk medicine practised in rural areas never actually went away under communism; some of these (e.g. herbalism in Bulgaria) are certainly flourishing (Fulder 1996:106).

Although there is considerable local variation, alternative medicines can no longer be regarded as marginal to the health care systems of western countries. In this book we wish to reflect on this movement from the margins by considering alternative medicine as a form of health care among many, as part of an overall field of health related activities – the social relations of health. This field includes not just the public and private services of doctors and the recognized paramedical professions, but also the services that "lay" people (especially women) provide for each other in the household, the many non-medical activities that people resort to in order to improve or maintain health (yoga, dieting, weight training, etc.) and of course the plurality of non-biomedical therapies which are the subject of this book.

What do we mean by pluralism?

Pluralism as a concept has been used in many different ways, most notably in relation to political phenomena. But we may agree with McLennan that "the force of any brand of pluralism depends on its ability to characterize and problematize some prevailing monistic orthodoxy" (McLennan 1995:98). Pluralism signals multiplicity, the interaction of a number of voices in any given arena, but following McLennan, we shall treat it as one of a pair of concepts; pluralism implies the possibility of some kind of "monism" and vice versa. There is otherwise the danger of using the concept in a way that begs the question of the distribution of power (as in the case of many uses of the term "multiculturalism").

This is evident if we consider the more specific concept of "medical pluralism". This idea was developed in the context of research on the countries of the South where a biomedical mo-nopoly of health care services has been the exception rather than the rule. Anthropological and sociological studies of sub-Saharan

3

Africa, Latin America, Asia and Melanesia have revealed much about the ways in which different kinds of healing systems exist alongside each other and interact with each other, also the ways in which sick people and their kin make decisions about what kind of healers to use. It is not possible to study biomedical health care in such areas without awareness of these other forms of healing, if only because few patients will ever use only one system of healing in their lives. Nonetheless, the "consumer" chooses among forms of healing that do not have equal prestige and accessibility. Healers differ in the degree of credibility and esteem they can command, and even though biomedicine is weakly developed in many countries of the South, it still bears an authority and prestige derived from various sources, not least its international dimension, its relationship with the state, and its perceived success in controlling certain life threatening conditions through modern drugs and technology.

So, while an ideal typical pluralism would suggest multiple players who compete on a level playing field, medical pluralism in the postcolonial world more usually represents a situation where such equality is only apparent. If there is a "new" medical pluralism in the West, how far does it resemble the pluralism sociologists and anthropologists have identified elsewhere? What new jostling for power is going on in the health care market? What range of different therapy groups are active today? Have they really acquired greater legitimacy, and is the orthodox medical profession experiencing a diminution of its hegemony, through forces of deprofessionalization, proletarianization and sheer unpopularity? Is a postmodern reading in order, one that speaks of plurality of language games and narratives, and of social practices treated as having equal validity? In short, is there equity, choice and genuine "pluralism" in the new picture, or just a revised division of labour? And if we are to describe this emergent situation as pluralism, what does this say about the possibilities of co-operation between alternative therapies and biomedicine?

Situating our work in terms of debates about pluralism does not mean that we think that what we see in western countries today is identical to that in postcolonial countries. (Our title is meant to be provocative rather than definitive.) But it does remind us that historically and geographically speaking, pluralism has been the norm rather than the exception. This being so, we shall need to question the assumption that has tended to dominate medical sociology in the West, namely that biomedicine must be the main focus of attention. This has meant that the contemporary study of other forms of healing has been located more in the field of the sociology of rejected knowledge than in the field of the sociology of health and healing. In this book we problematize this marginalization and propose new ways of studying alternative medicines.

Problems of scope and definition

What healing modes constitute "alternative medicine" – and is "alternative medicine" the best name for them? In this book we use the term "alternative medicine" to refer to forms of healing that depend on knowledge bases distinct from that of biomedicine and which, as such, do not share the special legitimation that the state has conferred upon biomedicine. Yet, non-biomedical modes of healing found in western countries are highly diverse and it can be argued that they should no longer be treated as a single category (Wardwell 1994:1062). Certainly, it is more proper to write of alternative *medicines* rather than alternative *medicine*.

For the most part these modes of healing are not new, but have their origins in various moments in the history of healing in the modern period. Most of them fall into one of five categories in terms of origins:

1) Those that developed prior to, or contemporaneously with, modern biomedicine. Among these we might include the various forms of phytotherapy, or herbalism, practised in Europe and America. Homoeopathy (developed in the early decades of the nineteenth century) also belongs in this group. In this rather heterogenous category we might also list various forms of unprofessionalized "folk" healing still found in some countries, such as cupping and bonesetting in Finland.

2) Those that originated in the period of medical individualism which characterized health care in America in the late nineteenth and early twentieth century, prior to the development of

tighter licensing laws and post-Flexner scientific medicine. Of these, chiropractic survived to become an extremely important component of the health care system in America and Canada. Osteopathy and radionics are other well known examples.

3) Those derived from the practices of central European health spas that flourished in the nineteenth century. Naturopathy, the best known form in this group, enjoyed a further florescence in the 1930s, when there was a wave of interest in health and fitness, outdoor pursuits and vegetarianism in Germany, and a number of other northern European countries.

4) Those that re-emerged in the West or were imported by westerners in various versions from Asia. The best known of these is probably acupuncture, but numerous other forms of oriental medicine have been imported to the West and "naturalized" there.

5) Those that have entered western countries with immigrant groups, such as Unani Tibb, Ayurveda and Chinese herbal medicine, not to mention various forms of ritual or "spiritual" healing or divining. Some of these are little known outside the ethnic groups who brought them, others have gained a wider repute and usage.

In as much as these forms of medicine have not been totally incorporated into biomedical practice and knowledge they do not share biomedicine's privileged relation to the state, though the precise nature and degree of their delegitimation varies from case to case and from country to country.

Rather than talk about the "rise" of alternative medicine in the past few decades it might be more accurate to speak, as Keith Bakx does, of its re-emergence after a period of "eclipse" (Bakx 1991). This eclipse commenced around the time at which organized biomedicine began to draw into a closer alliance with (on the one hand) the state and (on the other) laboratory science, i.e. around the end of the nineteenth century in most western countries. However, as many of the forms of non-biomedical healing that existed at that time never actually went away, it is quite hard to prove the exact scale of the modern re-emergence of alternative medicine. Another problem is that what lies "inside" or "outside" biomedicine at any one time is not always easy to decide. Healing modes like homoeopathy and acupuncture are widely practised by doctors in some countries, and some therapies (as we shall see) have a degree of legitimacy and standing with doctors such that describing them as "non-biomedical" might be regarded as contentious. One way of dealing with the terminological dilemma is simply to refer to "non-conventional" forms of healing. This is the usage preferred by the European Union (Lannoye 1996) and has the merit of avoiding judgements about the political place of these medicines. But it carries the same disadvantages as the term "non-biomedical" if we do not specify what degree of recognition is required for a form of medicine to be regarded as "conventional".

Similar problems attend the term "unorthodox" which can be used to refer to forms of healing within the biomedical camp that are regarded by the biomedical establishment as out of line or unscientific (Wolpe 1990). Biomedicine itself is not an undifferentiated entity (as medical anthropologists and sociologists constantly need to remind each other) and includes many voices (Atkinson 1995).

The term "unofficial" medicine is also useful, in as much as it conveys the sense of exclusion from the privileged authorization of state recognition. But whereas biomedicine is everywhere privileged by the state, the precise manner of that privileging, and hence the manner in which other forms of healing are disprivileged, is highly various. We deal with the typology of national health care systems in another chapter, but we should bear in mind for the moment that there is a range of types, from the "tolerant" position of the British state (where no form of healing is banned provided that its practitioners do not call themselves doctors), to the "exclusive" systems such as France and a number of other European countries, where any form of healing that is not part of the recognized repertoire of the medical doctor is illegal. The therapies we have in mind, therefore, occupy a variety of statutory positions in western countries.

As if all this complexity were not enough, the terminologies available to the social scientist are politically contentious for the healers themselves. In Britain, the term "alternative medicine" predominated in popular usage up to the end of the 1980s, implying associations with "alternative" lifestyles. As greater acceptance by doctors (even convergence with biomedicine) became apparent the term "complementary" came to be more widespread, signifying the possibility of a more co-operative relationship with biomedicine. This was a contentious issue among the therapists themselves; the use of the term "alternative" was held by many to indicate faithfulness to the idea that these healing modes were complete systems in their own right, whereas "complementary" indicated acceptance of a more limited position, subordinate to biomedicine. One way of avoiding this dilemma was to use terms like "natural" therapies (Inglis & West 1983).

In the United States of America the non-biomedical therapies were until recently commonly referred to as "holistic" healing. The use of this term now appears to us confusing since there is (in the USA and elsewhere) a version of biomedicine that claims to be holistic – its practitioners tend to be sympathetic to alternative medicines but do not necessarily practice them (for example, the model represented by the Maisons Médicales in francophone Belgium, Gobin 1984). Holism can be understood as the taking into account of the whole person and context of the patient, which could be a characteristic of many modes of healing – biomedical or otherwise. Most of the modes designated as alternative or complementary probably would claim to be holistic, but some are certainly more holistic than others and the claim to holism is not always understood in the same way. In the USA the term "alternative medicine" has recently come to be more widely used, and this is also the case where European writers publish in the English language. In a number of European countries the most commonly used local term is one that translates into English as " alternative" medicine. There are, however, some other very attractive possibilities. In French there is the term "*médicines douces*" (gentle medicines) also a German equivalent – "*sanfte Medizin*". There is also the term "*médicines parallèles*", referring to another possible positioning in relation to biomedicine.

Struggling to find an appropriate term, we realized that the indeterminacy of the field was a basic aspect of the very problem we set out to investigate. "Alternative medicine" (or more properly medicines) is at best a fluctuating and heterogeneous category, incapable of being sharply and universally demarcated from other forms of healing, or at least not in a way that is immediately applicable to the range of national situations. It is also a negative and formal category (that which is *not* biomedicine) rather than a substantive one.

In the end we decided that, since no term is without problems or objections, we would use the conventional and internationally understood term "alternative medicine" in the general context and when making international comparisons. However, we also use the terms "complementary medicines/therapies" when discussing Britain since these have become the more conventional terms there, and it seemed counter-intuitive to do otherwise.

These terms are widely understood, whatever their faults, and seem preferable to a social scientific neologism of our own which would probably be equally unsatisfactory from some point of view or another. Their use is not intended to imply any overall position about the degree of self-sufficiency of these diverse therapies or their possible relationship to biomedicine, present or future. Nor should the reader infer anything in particular from our use of the terms "medicines" and "therapies". The medical profession tends to refer to these modes as "therapies" and this would seem to be appropriate to the limited claims of some of them. Others are regarded by at least some of their proponents as complete systems of medicine, but we cannot take sides on this issue when we are writing in general terms.

Finally, we should note that in using the term "biomedicine" we are also using a term conventionally current among social scientists and wish to imply nothing in particular about the unity or coherence of this body of knowledge and treatment. The terms "cosmopolitan" medicine, "allopathy", "conventional" medicine and – in many European countries – "school" medicine are also widely used.

Medical sociology and alternative medicine: what might a sociological account of alternative medicine look like?

It must be descriptive, yet will go beyond the interpretive accounts already offered by participants in the field under review. If no-one still seriously believes that we can offer the objectivist "view from nowhere" (Bordo 1990: 143), it is surely possible to provide accounts that transcend the projects of what we have called the "players in the field". In the case of alternative medicine we are dealing with an area where differences in outlook have sometimes been profound, and conflicting claims bitterly debated. If sociologists cannot offer a view that is untainted by professional or any other kind of interest, then they can at least contextualize the various claims and positions in terms of wider social, political and economic processes.

But this very contextualization often assumes a unilinear periodization of social change which we wanted to avoid. When studying health and illness sociologists have tended to take the modernist project of biomedicine as their starting point, with the result that alternative medicine is liable to be characterized as either a "traditional" (premodern) survival (Sharma 1993) or potential herald of postmodernity (Bakx 1991). In taking the analysis of "what is going on" in a particular field beyond the self-evident we need to avoid the uncritical application of theoretical characterizations that are too broad to answer the question we are asking.

Many of these characterizations (preindustrial/industrial/ postindustrial, traditional/modern/postmodern) not only suggest unilinearity but are often applied by sociologsts in an ethnocentric way. Too often it is implied that what is happening in advanced industrial societies somehow stands for what is going on (or will be going on in the future) everywhere else. For example, as one (black) writer has remarked:

> Many of the writers of post-modernity have been very clear that only the "most highly developed societies" can be a party to the post-modern condition. This position is not just peculiar to Lyotard: it is also shared by Giddens and Rorty, among others. As a consequence the literature on postmodernity has a tendency to replay the modernist narrative. That is, the West preserves its vanguard role as the incarnation of the post-modern while the "Rest" get relegated to being just modern. (Sayyid 1997:111)

A sociological account of the re-emergence of alternative medicine is bound to concentrate on what is happening in the West, because (in the way we have formulated the question, at least) it is a western phenomenon. But there is no need for us to assume that what happens in the "Rest" is of purely archaeological interest. We shall take as global a view as is possible and make relevant cross-cultural comparisons.

How far will such an account say anything that is new, anything that is not already implied in the history of biomedical hegemony? Biomedicine is after all one of the most powerful "players" in the field we wish to study. Where sociologists are concerned, characterizations of medical hegemony have emerged from at least three strands of research. First, there is historical work that traces the emergence of biomedicine as a powerful way of knowing about the body and describes the rise of a medical profession privileged by the state (e.g. Larkin 1983, Stacey 1988). Recently, the influence of Foucault has informed much of this work, a Foucauldian perspective permitting the medical power to be considered in a broader context than that provided by the sociology of the professions. Medical power could now be understood in terms of the exercise of "biopower", and medical practice in terms of modern forms of the surveillance of populations, an emanation of governmentality (Lupton 1995:6).

A second strand is the tradition of micro-studies of the biomedical clinic which exposes the ways in which doctors are able to control talk and interaction in such a way that the "voice of medicine", as Mishler calls it, marginalizes the "voice of the lifeworld". Doctors may sometimes draw on shared discourses but their capacity to define the situation in the course of interaction with patients and with each other is still a dominant theme (e.g. Mishler 1984).

A third strand of research takes a step back from the clinic itself and asks how and why more and more areas of life come to be "medicalized" in the first place, i.e. defined as matters for the biomedical clinic. Thus infertility, alcoholism, mental disturbance, infant care (Wright 1988), even school refusal (Lock 1988), not to mention general unhappiness, came to be understood as quasi-sickness, problems for which interventions on the part of doctors are appropriate rather than those of, say, kin or priests.

The biomedical power which social scientists have wished to critique is no illusion. Historically speaking it has grown from (on the one hand) biomedicine's political alliance with the state and (on the other) its espousal of scientific method as the basis for its authoritative claims to knowledge and expertise.

The alliance with the state has taken different forms in different countries. Where the state is a major provider of health care services doctors have great power as gatekeepers to these services and the state may provide considerable support to medical training and research. Even where this is not the case, doctors generally constitute an insider group in the sense that their views and concerns are privileged by government (see Ch. 5). It is primarily scientific biomedical understandings of sickness and health that governments draw upon when they attempt to exercise surveillance and control over the bodies of citizens.

The espousal of scientific method has meant that the dominant forms of medical knowledge are those which present themselves as constituted according to experimental and investigative methods that have great social prestige. More than this, they allow doctors to claim both objectivity and rationality when they make clinical judgments which, in their effects, are often also moral judgements (what is and is not organic illness? what procedures do or do not cure? which patients should or should not be treated? what is the likely prognosis of a condition like ME?).

As a consequence of these alliances the medical profession in western countries has acquired great powers of disposal over patients – even where, as in the USA, biomedical health care is organized on market principles and not funded directly by the state. It has to a great extent been doctors who have in one way or another defined the modern role of other healing professions. Biomedicine's alliance with the state automatically marginalized other forms of healing where it did not actually render them illegitimate. In some countries professional medical organizations have ruled that doctors should not co-operate with non-biomedical healers.

Within the biomedical clinic, the medical profession has presided over the division of healing labour (Freidson 1970:47ff), with groups like nurses, physiotherapists, dieticians, etc. positioned in relation to the doctor in the clinic and drawing very heavily on medical knowledge in the technical aspects of their work. (This is a very broad generalization since this positioning has varied greatly from state to state, and some groups – such as midwives – have often resisted it vigorously. See, for example, Witz 1992.)

Until now this division of labour has either excluded entirely or provided only a very limited place for alternative practitioners who are not also doctors themselves. It is true that in many countries certain forms of alternative medicine can be practised in the bio-

medical clinic by qualified doctors. There are also important exceptions such as the German heilpraktiker, who are licensed by the
state to practice a form of "nature cure" with hydrotherapy, and
who need not be medical doctors. There is also the curiously protected role of homoeopathy in the British National Health Service
(NHS), a relic of homòeopathy's former popularity among a section
of medical doctors, also possibly a reflection of its continued popularity with the British royal family. A major contemporary problem
for alternative medicines, as we shall see, is whether or not the
professions wish to accept some such positioning – giving them a
secure position in the official health care system, but one defined for
them in terms of the biomedical division of labour.

In the light of such considerations, the notion of medical hegemony is a realistic and convincing one, which we shall certainly
need to draw upon in our analysis of alternative medicines.

On the other hand, a sociological problematic that privileges the
biomedical clinic may lead to other sites of healing activity being
overlooked. For instance, it is now recognized that the sociology of
health and healing must include a consideration of the ways in which
the work of lay carers (especially women) in the home contributes to
the production of health (Stacey 1988:206). Other areas which are
still insufficiently studied might include the role of pharmacists and
other high street sellers of remedies, health foods, etc. In Britain, the
assumption on the part of medical sociologists that pluralism is not
an issue and that the state funded biomedical clinic should be the
main focus for their research has had the consequence that the
medical market place in general has been neglected as a object of
study – even the private biomedical clinic has been little studied
(with a few exceptions such as Higgins 1988, Calnan et al. 1993, also
Bennett et al. 1997).

Taking for granted the hegemony and pre-eminence of biomedicine has not entirely precluded studies of alternative medicine.
There has been research on particular therapies in a number of
countries, and of holistic clinics in the USA (Mattson 1982:92). But
to our mind a major problem with much of this is that it has been
positioned as research "on the margins". Alternative medicines
have been studied largely in terms of discredited knowledge,
marginal medicine (e.g. Gevitz 1988a). Social scientists, in spite of

themselves, have taken on the "meta-narrative" of biomedicine about its rise and universalism, albeit without the triumphalism of medicine's own account of itself.

This being so, analytical studies (in the English language literature at least) have looked at alternative medicines first and foremost in terms of the nature and progress of claims made by their practitioners and the ways in which these were received by the biomedical establishment. There has been less focus on issues such as how therapies recruit practitioners, what goes on in the alternative practitioner's clinic (though see Oths 1994, Johannessen 1996), the ways in which patients understand their claims and procedures. Only recently have writers such as Coward (1989) revisited the issues originally raised by Crawford (1980) and examined holism and alternative medicine as indicative of broad cultural change, of novel transformations of central concerns about the body, health and individual responsibility.

What we intend to do in this study is to give due importance to the crucial role of biomedical dominance in determining the position of alternative medicines in the present century without seeing them entirely through a biomedical lens. Even sociologists who have confined their study to biomedicine are now asking questions about the possibility of a demedicalization of society, a deprofessionalization or even proletarianization of doctors. Medical power itself is no longer regarded by sociologists as constant and unproblematic and some have focused on the various challenges to biomedicine that stem from the greater "consumer" awareness (even litigiousness) of patients, widespread anxieties about side effects of drugs, the presence of alternative healing practices, and many other factors (Elston 1991, Gabe et al. 1994a). Taking medical power seriously without taking it for granted means that we will avoid the assumption that biomedicine and alternative medicines are involved in some kind of zero sum power contest; we can see both of them as embedded in a wider field of power relations.

What is the field and who are the players?

This wider context may be termed the "social relations of health". We look on the production of health (whatever that is taken to mean in a given society) as a field of activity that may involve various persons and agencies. These would obviously include persons explicitly defined as sick or as actively seeking to maintain their health, their carers or responsible kin, healing practitioners of all kinds, other occupational groups whose work has directly or indirectly to do with the production of health such as nurses, health visitors and hospital chaplains. Other important agencies would include the state, to the extent that the state regulates the provision of health care or is actually a provider itself; pharmaceutical companies and other makers or purveyors of medicines and remedies; insurance companies (in as much as these validate claims for health care made against insurance policies); and educators and informers – both those with an explicit remit to promote health, but also others for whom health is only one aspect of their work (such as school teachers, journalists).

The advantage of this perspective is that it makes no assumptions about the degree to which such relations can be conceived as a system; the agencies concerned may engage with each other through many different modes of conjunction – statutory, domestic, professional – and there need not be consistency or agreement about such engagements. For example, a major issue which we shall discuss is the debate about whether alternative medicine in Britain should be subject to regulation by the state or whether it should be organized according to market principles. Another problematic area is the issue of how far and in what way GPs need to be informed about alternative treatments being received by their patients.

In this book we give accounts of alternative medicines from four selected (but important) points of view – those of users, of alternative practitioners, of doctors and of governments – represented schematically in the diagram on the next page. These "key players" have interests that are at times conflicting, at others intertwined, engaging with each other in a field which is bounded by broad (and changing) "climates" of thinking about health and the body, about the responsibilities of doctors, citizens and governments for the health of individuals and collectivities. Diagram 1 is an attempt to represent these relationships in a rough and ready and (no doubt) incomplete way. We have tried to indicate the engagement of the key players with each other and with other groups or agencies.

15

Diagram 1: Key players in the development of alternative medicine

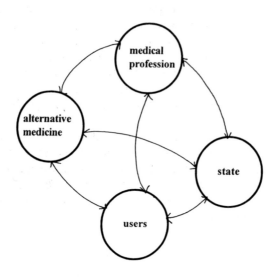

We hope to demonstrate how such a widening of the context in which the issue of alternative medicines is considered leads to a better sociological understanding of their importance. As a preview of the structure of the book, we will briefly consider the kinds of questions that we need to ask about the four sets of players which we have identified.

Users

The literature on medical pluralism in the postcolonial world focuses very largely on the consumers of health care and the processes by which they make their decisions (how do sick people in Ivory Coast, Papua New Guinea or India choose which kind of healer to consult? which ones are preferred for which kinds of problem? (e.g. Strathern 1989). Medical sociologists in the West have tended to assume that the critical user decision to be studied is whether or not to consult a doctor, so we know rather little about how people make decisions about alternative medicines. The considerable survey literature on users' reasons for using a particular form of alternative medicine is restricted by its methodology and does not tell us very much about process. That is, it tells us quite a lot about what sort of people use alternative medicines and the reasons they give for a particular consultation, but has less to say about how usage might be derived from or even bring about broad changes in ideas about health and illness or expectations about what doctors and healers can deliver.

We shall need to pay more attention to cultural process, asking how far use of alternative medicines is seen in terms of consumer choice. If usage is on the increase, is this related to changing attitudes to the body, to personal responsibility for health, to the role of biomedicine in producing health? How might such changes be related to other cultural changes?

Alternative practitioners

Here a major concern must be the extent to which these healers constitute professionalized groups and the ways in which such groups have emerged. We shall ask how these groups have seen their position – what kind of positioning within the social relations of health have they sought, and by what means have they sought it? How far have they been able or willing to pursue radical projects, how far have they either chosen or been obliged to accept a degree of convergence with biomedicine? Most existing studies relate to groups that have developed a degree of professional organization, but we must always remember that there are many people who earn a living through healing work who are not professionalized to any great degree (e.g. some spiritual healers, some healers from ethnic minorities).

Biomedicine

Notwithstanding what we have said about medical sociologists' over-concentration on the relationship between alternative medicines and biomedicine, we shall need to look at doctors' responses to the knowledge claims of alternative practitioners and to the fact that doctors are not the only source of authority about health and illness for many of their patients. We shall look at the collective responses of the medical profession expressed through professional organizations, but also the ways in which such responses relate to the attitudes and activities of individual doctors, some of whom practice forms of alternative medicine themselves. Are there signs of a softening of either individual or collective medical attitudes and, if so, is this simply due to changed perceptions of professional self-interest? Or is there a shift towards more holistic understandings of the doctor's (especially the GP's) role, perhaps a greater acceptance of patients' demands for participation?

The state

In as much as states vouchsafe the privileged position of biomedicine, we need to examine governmental attitudes to alternative medicines. There is a range of ways in which states attempt to order relations among health care professionals – ranging from those that outlaw any practice other than biomedicine to those who are inclined to leave more to a medical market, with the state having only a regulatory role. We need to ask about directions of and reasons for any change in governmental attitudes (in response to what pressures?). If there is some softening of governmental attitudes in many countries, is this related to broader political trends, for example the tension between regulatory and deregulatory tendencies in western countries, the widespread revision of welfare provision and state expenditure?

Encompassing concerns

The social relations of health are, in turn, embedded in encompassing social and cultural relations, and we shall attempt to relate the changes we document to wider sociological issues of contemporary concern.

For instance, it has often been suggested that biomedicine is of its nature particularly suited to serve the needs of capitalism. It is a "core institution of capitalist society and . . . a system that reinforced dominance at the micro-social level" (Singer & Baer 1995:62). If this is so, do alternative medicines represent some kind of counter-culture or resistance? Or can alternative medicines themselves be co-opted to a role in the control of populations? Can holism (with its stress on individual responsibility) become a latter day practice of self-surveillance? (Berliner & Salmon 1980:548–9, Kotarba 1983, Coward 1989, Braathen 1996). Does this individualistic approach carry the danger of encouraging sick people to feel personal responsibility for conditions that are patently not a product of their own actions, but of general social or environmental conditions (Kopelman & Moskop 1981)?

Diagram 2: Alternative medicine and the wider social context

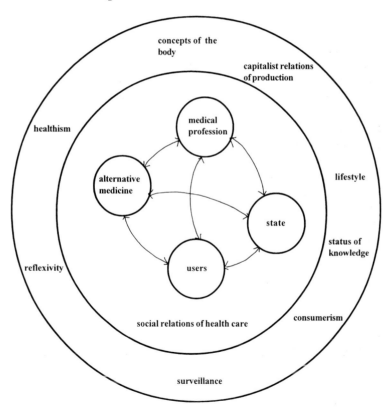

Perhaps we should see alternative medicines as a dimension of the reflexive nature of high modernity as defined by Giddens (Giddens 1991:74ff), with their stress on self-monitoring and the confessional nature of certain kinds of holistic consultation? What does an examination of alternative medicines tell us about the role of expert knowledge and professionals in modern societies and the extent of trust in what Giddens calls "abstract systems"? Does increased usage of alternative medicines represent a destabilization of biomedicine and science as forms of knowledge? If so, should we regard the resurgence of non-biomedical forms of healing as an instance of postmodern rejection of universalism, a fragmentation of the authority of the medical meta-narrative?

We should be looking for such shifts in the constitution of civil society and in the behaviour of states, for our account will be pedestrian if we do not address these issues. In the light of these totalizing concerns we could redraw our diagram of the geography of our field to represent the enfolding of our four key groups within a wider cultural context.

In defining the field broadly we want to build on what we learnt from our previous research on the professionalization of alternative medicines, namely that "what is going on" is a product of interaction among a plurality of actors, that there is in a sense no simple history of alternative medicine (Cant & Sharma 1996a), or none that can be told without innumerable qualifications and variations. There are different stories of different medicines told from various perspectives. However we hope that in this book we can experiment with an account that is inclusive without being either vacuous or ethnocentric, integrating as many of these perspectives as proves possible.

CHAPTER 2

The nature of user demand: from patient to consumer?

The popularity of alternative medicine is not difficult to demonstrate. A quick scan of the health section in the local bookshop, the array of remedies available at the chemist, the regular inclusion of articles in newspapers and women's magazines or an analysis of the content of television programmes provide ample anecdotal evidence even before we examine the wealth of survey material that has been generated and which details the number of users and their socio-demographic characteristics (e.g. MORI 1989, Thomas et al. 1991). But what motivates people to choose alternative medicine, to potentially contradict the advice of their general practitioner, to undergo treatment that has not been submitted to rigorous scientific testing and, in many countries, reach into their own pockets to pay for services that stand outside health care that is funded by the state? What decisions are involved and how do the patients actually use the services? Have they exited from biomedicine altogether or do they use alternative and biomedical services simultaneously? And does this shift in purchasing decisions point to deeper social and cultural changes relating to the body, understandings of health and illness and the belief in science? Perhaps the story is a simple one, that patients have become more discerning and discontented, have higher incomes and expectations. The purchase of health care possibly mirrors the purchase of a car or a new sofa, the consumer looking for the best buy and the most amenable salesperson. What is certain is that there has been a significant change in the behaviour of users of health care and the only way to try to answer these questions is to turn to an investigation of their views, beliefs and expectations.

The importance of lay health beliefs[1] has long been recognized within medical sociology, in particular that lay people do not simply accept biomedical definitions of health and illness or indeed what is appropriate illness behaviour. On the contrary, the lay public hold alternative, complex yet rational ideas about health and illness that interact with biomedical knowledge. The acknowledgement of culturally and socially located definitions of health and illness that have an impact upon health related behaviour has generated a range of research questions that have relevance for an understanding of alternative medicine. Until the late 1970s (Nettleton 1995, Bury 1997), research tended to focus upon and provide insightful commentary on patterns of help seeking behaviour, lay referral and the consumption of health services, revealing examples of under and over utilization (Hannay 1979, Cartwright & Anderson 1981). It became clear that decisions about appropriate health care were mediated by cultural understandings of health and illness and local social networks (Zborowski 1952, Zola 1973, Freidson 1970). Investigations into the nature of *health* beliefs and ideas about causation and susceptibility to illness (rather than illness behaviour) have also revealed that lay peoples hold complex and often apparently contradictory views[2] (Herzlich 1973, Calnan 1987). In particular, people tend to relate their illness experience to life events (Cornwell 1984) and do not simply accept that poor health is the product of the operation of objective pathogens. More practically, investigations into the influence of lifestyles have proven invaluable to the understanding of health promotion activity (Pill & Stott 1982, Davison et al. 1992). Thus, Herzlich (1973) argued that her sample of middle-class people conceived of health as internal to the individual and believed in each individual's capacity to maintain good health whereas, in contrast, other research has shown that working-class people tend to have less positive conceptions of health and are less likely to engage in preventative programmes (Pill & Stott 1982). The product of this research has been to show that lay beliefs are not only complex but rational and are influential in determining health and illness behaviour.

A second important strand of research has revealed how illness episodes (particularly those associated with chronic illness) shape the sufferer's identity, experiences and sense of self (Bury 1997). This should not be conceived as deterministic. Drawing on·

interactionist perspectives, sociologists have shown that individuals actively make sense of their illness. For example, sufferers of chronic illness need explanations about why *they* have become ill. Biomedical explanations about the causes of illness are never sufficient, instead more meaning is drawn when illness can be tied to the individual's own biography and through the re-interpretation of past life events (Williams 1984). In other words, substantial work has revealed the importance of imputing and gaining meaning from illness episodes. Thus, the lay public draw on socially and culturally available categories (which have their own logic and validity), from personal and family stories, to make their experiences meaningful and use this information to re-interpret their lives, identity and relationships. The human capacity to respond to illness, to give it meaning and use the experience to re-order one's own understanding of the social world and one's place in it is nothing new, but it is pertinent to ask whether alternative medicine draws more explicitly upon such repertoires than biomedicine.

Turning our attention to the study of the patient also raises interesting historical parallels. Jewson (1976) describes how the production of medical knowledge changed between 1770 and 1870 and the implications this had for the doctor–patient relationship. With bedside medicine, the patient chose and paid for the services they desired, care was patient centred and the doctor was relatively powerless. This form of health care was replaced as medicine became more scientific (moving from hospital to laboratory medicine), patients' views and explanations of their disease became less important and care became distinctly doctor centred. To what extent can the increased popularity of alternative medicine be seen to be a challenge to this balance of power, especially as alternative practitioners claim to put the patient centre stage (Johannessen 1996)? Have we moved full circle, with the patient treated less as a bundle of cells and more as a person who can have a say over their health care programme? Specifically, have we seen the traditional patient of health care also becoming a "consumer", choosing the services they desire and seeing themselves as active decision makers? Stacey (1976) has argued that within the National Health Service it is a misconception to view the patient as a consumer because the relationship between doctor and patient can be exploitative and the patient takes a position of work object for the doctor. Does the

23

process of help seeking within the alternative medical sector alter this position of powerlessness?

The "consumption" of health care has, of course, been encouraged by recent government policy in Britain which favours contractual relations between doctors and patients and has stipulated that the consumer be at the centre of health policy decisions (DOH 1989a, 1991). Consumerism in this context tends to mean the maximization of consumer choice, provision of information, reduced waiting times, encouraging consumers to complain and taking consumers' views into account by conducting surveys to ascertain satisfaction levels (Nettleton 1995). This has coincided with wider social and cultural change (see Bakx 1991) that sociologists expect will work to equalize the relationship between the consumer and providers of health care. Specifically, raised reflexivity and knowledgeability on the part of the patient coupled with the increased distrust of expert knowledge (Giddens 1990, Beck 1992) may provide for a situation where the relationship between the patient and practitioner may change.

The lessons from previous studies of the lay public and the changing social, political and cultural environment suggest important research questions regarding the alternative medical sector. In particular, which groups actually "consume" these services: are they more discerning and knowledgeable, are they distrustful of biomedicine? This chapter takes the user as its focus in an attempt to examine in more detail the shape and nature of the new medical pluralism. Holding multiple understandings of what facilitates health and causes disease would suggest a form of pluralism. But to what extent is this new? If previous studies have taught us anything it is that patients hold a complex and often contradictory set of ideas about health and illness (Stacey 1988). However, if these views encourage using a mix of services, a more critical stance towards the medical experts and a shift from patient to consumer then there has been a shift in behaviour and attitude.

Theorizing consumption of alternative medicine

Before we examine the empirical data that has been generated about the users of alternative medicine, is it possible to draw any

24

insight from the wealth of theoretical material that has been generated within sociology about recent social change? Certainly it is clear that a number of critical changes are occurring in what has variously been described as late, radical or post-modernity, changes that carry implications for the way that biomedicine is perceived and the role of the lay public as consumers of health care. Where the expansion of scientific knowledge promised progress and predictability, it can be suggested that instead there have been unforeseen and unwelcome consequences associated with the expansion of knowledge (Giddens 1990), notably risks, and in the case of medicine concerns, about side effects associated with many biomedical interventions. It is generally agreed that the general public have become increasingly sceptical about the value of medicine (Gabe et al. 1994a) but has there been a fracturing of societal trust? Of course, there can never have been complete trust but has the faith in the medical profession declined and are users of alternative medicine more sceptical and concerned about biomedicine? Bakx (1991) has argued that biomedicine has lost the support of the lay public:

> biomedicine is in danger of losing both its actual and ideological hegemony: firstly, it has culturally distanced itself from the consumers of its services; secondly it has failed to match its propaganda polices with real breakthroughs; thirdly patients have become further alienated by negative physical and psychological experiences at the hands of the biomedical practitioners themselves. (Bakx 1991:33)

The questioning of science and of the experts that have translated the scientific knowledge (in this case, doctors) cannot have occurred without an increase in the knowledgeability of the lay public. Giddens (1990, 1991) suggests that the lay public are increasingly informed and reflexive, especially as knowledge has become pluralized. In such a context it is likely, Giddens argues, that individuals, communities and institutions will attempt to "re-skill" – by wresting back some control from the "experts" and by searching for alternatives. There is evidence that the lay public have increasingly endeavoured to re-appropriate knowledge for themselves (e.g. Oakley 1984, Williams & Popay 1994) and perhaps the turning to alternative medicine could be seen as part of that re-skilling process? Interestingly, research about users of private health insurance

(Calnan et al. 1993) established that the consumers were not particularly knowledgeable about health care and did not exhibit active
involvement in decision making about the choice of hospital or
consultant. However, in Britain, private health services are mediated by the state funded general practitioner and it is possible that
alternative medicine, still largely separate from general practice,
may offer new and different opportunities.

Certainly, it is widely agreed that users of alternative medicine
desire more from their relationship with their practitioners, in particular that they be more involved in the healing process. The practitioner–patient relationship within alternative medicine can be very
different to that found within the biomedical clinic (Johannessen
1996), and Taylor (1984) has suggested that it is dissatisfaction with
the medical encounter and the hierarchical and disempowering
modes of consultation within biomedicine that explains the popularity of alternative medicine. Here we find some parallels with the
private medical sector in the United Kingdom as empirical research
has shown that users of private medical services are attracted by the
extra time they are given by the private doctor and the changes this
can facilitate in the doctor–patient relationship, although it is often
the speed in which a patient can see a consultant rather than the
length of time spent in the consulting room which is most desired
(Higgins 1988, Calnan et al. 1993, Wiles & Higgins 1996). Moreover,
patients within the private sector often characterize the relationship
as one of friendship and argue that they feel more assertive in their
dealings with their doctor (Wiles & Higgins 1996). The relationship
between the alternative medical practitioner and the user may also
be radically different, offering a more personal approach that is
concentrated on the whole person.

Within sociology the interest in the process and meaning of
consumption has also escalated in the last ten years. The consumption of goods and services is recognized as a socio-cultural process
(Bocock 1993) that is now regarded as having more impact upon the
identity and lifestyle of a person than production (Saunders 1988),
although there is much evidence to suggest a continued and strong
link between consumption and a person's social and economic
position (Charles & Kerr 1988, Calnan et al. 1993). The increased
emphasis given to consumption, its cultural meaning and the range
of available consumable goods has also been linked, alongside the

importance of self reflexivity, to concerns about the maintenance ᴜɪ the body. Featherstone (1991) has thus talked about the commercialization of healthy lifestyles and both Giddens (1991) and Shilling (1993) talk of the "body project" whereby people increasingly see the body as an unfinished project to be shaped by lifestyle choices. Indeed Shilling, drawing on Giddens, suggests that in times of risk and uncertainty, the body becomes a site where individuals can exert control:

> Investing in the body project provides people with a means of self expression and a way of potentially feeling good and increasing the control that they have over their bodies. (Shilling 1993: 7)

Are users of alternative medicine more concerned about their "healthy bodies" than non-users? Ros Coward (1989) has linked the use of alternative medicine to the wider shift in expectations about health care, particularly "healthism", the cultivation of a highly individualistic approach to the body which emphasizes not just the perfectibility of the body, but the right of the individual to attain such perfect health and the obligation and responsibility of every individual to pursue such perfectibility.

Of course the consumption of healthy lifestyles, like any consumption, must be constrained by social and material resources. Consumption taste and decisions have been shown to be socially distributed and the application of Bourdieu's (1984) concept of "distinction" to middle-class consumption patterns, for example, showed that consumption of different health related goods had become a distinguishing feature of social position (Savage et al. 1992). Furthermore, work by Bunton & Burrows (1995) was able to draw a link between the rise in consumer culture and health promotion activity but only in the middle classes. Is it possible to discern such differences among users of alternative medicine?

Examining the views of users of alternative medical services thus allows us to ask highly significant questions about what motivates people to change their consumption patterns. Are there differences in the beliefs and values of the users, are they more concerned about risks of biomedical intervention and are they more reflexive about their health and their bodies? Is this a change that is peculiar to particular social groups and does it therefore say something about lifestyle and income? What do the users expect and how educated were they about the practice? The remainder of this chapter reviews the empirical evidence to try and shed some light on these questions. Our analysis is somewhat constrained by the nature of the studies thus far conducted which contain a number of methodological problems. First, most studies take users as their focus and do not make comparisons with non-users and as such it is often difficult to make generalized conclusions. Secondly, even if we use qualitative methods there are huge difficulties in studying decision-making when one is trying to unpick the way that some decisions have been made in retrospect. After all, to examine the point of choice is to isolate a moment in what is often an ongoing story of attempts to deal with illness and accounts will change with greater experience of the practitioner, the progress of the illness, etc. In other words, we must acknowledge that the account of resort to an alternative medical practitioner is part of an "illness narrative" (Kleinman 1988, Good 1994). Thirdly, quantitative surveys vary tremendously in terms of the question posed. For example, some ask respondents whether they have ever used alternative medicine while others ask about use in the last year. These differences make comparisons difficult.

How extensive is the demand for alternative medicine?

Survey data suggests that there is considerable interest in alternative medicine and that the numbers of consumers of these services continues to grow. In the United Kingdom, for instance, *WHICH?*[3] conducted three surveys of its readers in 1986, 1992 and 1995. It is difficult to generalize from this data as it was constructed from replies to a readers' questionnaire, and so it is possible that those people that used alternative medical services may have been more inclined to fill in the questionnaire. Nevertheless, it is possible to compare the three studies and to chart changes in consumption within this particular group. In the first survey, one in seven members claimed to have used some form of alternative medical practice and this almost doubled by 1992 to one in four (25 per cent) and by 1995 was one in three. This figure has been supported by regional studies funded by health authorities in Britain (see Emslie et al. 1996).

Although there are some differences when we compare countries, and quantifying use is difficult because of the differences in survey instrument and population coverage, a figure of 20–25 per cent seems to be consistent and in some cases modest. In the United States, a national study found that 34 per cent of the sample had used at least one therapy in the last year (Eisenberg et al. 1993). In Australia, 20.3 per cent of a sample of 3,004 respondents had visited one practitioner in the last year (MacLennan et al. 1996). Elsewhere in Europe similar figures are available, for example, in Holland 21.6 per cent of the population had seen an alternative practitioner or their doctor for alternative therapy (Menges 1994) and in Belgium, Finland and France, approximately one-third of people have had some form of alternative medical treatment in the last twelve months (Lewith & Aldridge 1991; also see Sermeus (1987) for a summary of nine European countries).

Who are the users?

Is the use of alternative medicine confined to a small group of wealthy and articulate people or is it, as according to popular mythology, a fringe activity undertaken by vegans who wear plastic shoes? Are users more neurotic or hypochondriacal than the average population? If the surveys are correct and at least a fifth of the population have used alternative medicine in the last year it suggests that this is not a marginal exercise. Moreover, data about the socio-demographic characteristics of users shows that they are very similar to the non-users. There are some differences in that users are more likely to be women (usually making up about two-thirds of the users), middle aged and middle class (RSGN 1984, MORI 1989, Thomas et al. 1991). This kind of data is consistent with that of researchers in other countries (for Europe see Sermeus 1987; Australia see Australian Bureau of Statistics 1992; America see Eisenberg et al. 1993). In other words there is no obvious "type" of user although a more recent study undertaken in Australia suggested that users came from a very select group with a narrow range of social demographic backgrounds (Lloyd et al. 1993), in particular they found that users were more likely to live alone, be university educated and covered by private health insurance and were less likely to smoke and drink alcohol. The authors concluded from these findings that users were more conscious about their health and concerned with healthy living.

Overall these differences need not be too surprising. The large number of women users may be related to the likelihood that they experience chronic illnesses more than men and their preparedness to consult the biomedical services more extensively. Yet this observation does not account for the statistical likelihood that they would have less disposable income than their male counterparts (Pahl 1989). However, it is also the case in Britain that men hold private health insurance policies but it is their wives who utilize the services (Calnan et al. 1993) and it is possible that a similar pattern exists for the alternative medical services. Certainly, the fact that users usually pay privately or use private health insurance means that the finding that users have higher incomes is not too revealing.

All British studies have shown that there are regional differences in use, the North of England and Scotland generally having much lower levels of consultation (MORI 1989) but this may reflect the greater number of practitioners and training schools in the South (Fulder & Munro 1982, Thomas et al. 1991). Certainly in our study of reflexologists, chiropractors and homoeopaths, it was noticeable that training schools were clustered in the South and that these attracted local students who then chose to practice in the same area. Even in the case of the largest college of chiropractic in Bournemouth (south coast of England), which attracts students from all over Europe, we found the highest concentration of chiropractors in this area (Cant & Sharma 1994). Considering, as we shall see later, that most patients make the decision to consult on the basis of recommendation, this suggests that it may be the supply of practitioners that encourages demand and the extent of usage may be greater if the number of practitioners were to increase and situate themselves in all parts of the country. In other words, the full extent of usage of these services may be artificially constrained.

This body of research has thus generated useful data about the socio-demographic characteristics of users but has largely failed to offer explanations about why people turn to alternative medicine in the first place, their patterns of use or whether there are variations in values, attitudes and beliefs held by users and non-users. More recently, a number of quantitative studies have sought to assess the extent to which there are differences in perceived susceptibility to disease, beliefs about self-control, attitudes to health promotion and views about the perceived efficacy of biomedical treatment. This work has largely been pioneered by Furnham who, with colleagues, has revealed a number of statistically significant differences between users and non-users, although these vary according to which therapy is studied. For example, users of homoeopathy were found to be more critical and sceptical of biomedicine (Furnham & Smith 1988, Furnham & Bragrath 1992) and were more conscious about their health generally. A further study in 1994 (Furnham & Forey 1994) revealed that the users of homoeopathy were also more likely to believe that their health could be improved and had more self and ecologically aware lifestyles, were concerned about ensuring a holistic approach to health care and were generally more knowledgeable about their bodies than patients who only used biomedicine. These findings have been replicated in Germany (Furnham & Kirkcaldy 1996) and start to offer some indications about the possible attractions of alternative medicine rather than the dissatisfactions of biomedicine. Nevertheless, some further differences appear when users of different therapies are studied. For example, a study of users of acupuncture (Furnham et al. 1995) revealed lower levels of confidence in GPs than non-users and a reduced faith in biomedical drugs. Such dissatisfaction was not revealed in the study of homoeopathic patients, although a study in America (Yu et al. 1994) showed homoeopathic patients to be more displeased with biomedicine than users of chiropractic. The important point is that there are differences among users of alternative medicine as much as differences between users and non-users. For example, when comparing users of osteopathy, homoeopathy and acupuncture (Vincent & Furnham 1996), homoeopathic patients were shown to value their involvement in the healing process to a far greater extent than the other users and the acupuncture users were the most concerned about the side effects of biomedical drugs. Such findings should caution us from making general statements about users of alternative medicine *per se* and encourage therapy specific analysis. Overall, this body of research has pointed to scepticism towards biomedicine at some levels and evidence that users may be more reflexive and conscious about their health status.

Popular therapies and patterns of care

What do we learn about usage if we examine which therapies are popular, the actual processes of help seeking and the manner in which consumers make the decision to use alternative medicine? It is estimated that there are at least 160 therapies available in the United Kingdom (BMA 1993) but this does not mean that they are all used equally or for the same reasons. On the contrary, studies in Britain and elsewhere have shown that it is a relatively small group of therapies that attract the most popular support (Sharma 1992, Fulder 1996), namely, acupuncture, homoeopathy, herbalism, osteopathy and chiropractic but it is also the case that reflexology and aromatherapy are experiencing greater support than before (Fulder & Munro 1982, NAHAT 1993, Fisher & Ward 1994). The support for these groups of therapies may be a reflection of the number of practitioners available in these disciplines, their public profile and the media coverage they receive, as well as their success in treatment but whatever the reason it means that the pluralistic use of services is confined to a fairly contained number of therapies. Such findings have been replicated in America, where it was shown that 10 per cent of a national sample had used one of only four therapies, namely chiropractic, relaxation therapy, acupuncture and therapeutic massage (Paramore 1997).

It is generally agreed that most patients attend for chronic rather than acute conditions, notably health problems where bio-medicine cannot offer a panacea (Cant & Calnan 1991, Sharma 1992). Sharma (1992) identified pain (especially back pain) and allergies as the most frequent presenting problems and certainly osteopaths and chiropractors are used extensively throughout the world for lower back pain (Thomas et al. 1991), this being the area that these practitioners have identified as their speciality (see Ch. 3 and Ch. 5). Acupuncture has been linked to the relief of chronic pain and migraines (Fulder 1996 – an area that the medical profession recognize as acupuncture's forte, see Ch. 4), whereas homoeopaths tend to see more non-specific conditions, allergies and stress related illness and diseases that relate to inadequate immunity. The association between chronic illness and alternative medicine may well reflect the fact that alternative practitioners claim to encourage patient participation and chronicity is an area where the patient can become very knowledgeable and desire inclusion in decision making (West 1976). However, these patterns may be exaggerated because most research studies take the more established therapies as their focus and they may also be specific to the United Kingdom. In Australia, for example, Lloyd et al. (1993) found in their more detailed study that musculo-skeletal conditions only accounted for a fifth of consultations and that there were a wide range of problems seen by alternative practitioners. The focus on these therapies tends to suggest that people are turning to alternative medicine for a cure, as a last resort for conditions where biomedicine has failed them.

If we turn our attention to the less used therapies we can identify different reasons for seeking such care. For instance, it is the case in Britain that reflexology does not make any public claims to offer cures (Cant & Sharma 1996a), instead the emphasis is upon relaxation and the enhancement of feelings of wellbeing for the patient. Similarly, many beauty treatments are included in the broader definitions of alternative medicine and they too are concerned with care rather than cure. Perhaps there has been a blurring of what kind of activity can be defined as "health care"? Consumers may not necessarily be unwell in a biomedical sense and consequently we may need to re-define what constitutes health related behaviour, the disease model now seemingly inadequate. Where health care has been equated with medical techniques of the body, it may now need to broaden to include all those recreational and aesthetic techniques that the consumer links to "feeling healthy". Nevertheless, the evidence that alternative medicine is concerned with intractable and chronic conditions seems undeniable.

Focusing on actual processes of help seeking behaviour reveals interesting patterns of usage. In the first place, the most overwhelming finding is that patients tend to see their biomedical practitioner before they seek care from the alternative practitioner and rarely abandon biomedical care in total (Thomas et al. 1991, Sharma 1992). In Holland (Ooijendijk et al. 1981) it was shown that the majority of users continued to see their general practitioner (85 per cent) with 32 per cent visiting their doctor between three and seven times a year and 22 per cent visiting eight times or more. That is, there was a significant category of people who were high users of both kinds of medicine. This raises important policy and financial questions about the pluralistic use of services. Does the use of alternative medicine lead to effective deployment of health budgets if patients also simultaneously use biomedicine? Certainly, it may please biomedical doctors that they are not abandoned and that they can continue to monitor the progress of their patients but in many cases patients are effectively receiving double amounts of care. Governments may then be cautious about bringing these services into state funded health care if the pressure on biomedicine is not relieved and there is no room to simply redeploy existing budgets. Lewisham Health Authority in England decided to stop funding alternative medical services in 1997 because of the cost to their budgets, and in Australia the government has resisted calls to include alternative medical services under its medicare scheme (Easthope 1993).

However, this broad brush characterization can be broken down further if we look at usage more carefully and it may be that all users are not so "draining" on health care. In Sharma's (1992) study in one Midland locality users were divided into three main types. The "earnest seekers" were those consumers who were prepared to try a variety of approaches for one condition and did not intend to carry on with alternative medicine once their immediate problem was resolved. Here, for instance, there was some evidence of users who simultaneously used herbal remedies and analgesics. "Stable users" had a regular relationship with a particular practitioner or therapy, and in this category it is possible that such a relationship may enable the users to consult their practitioner more regularly and without always also consulting their general practitioner. "Eclectic users" were those consumers that shopped around among practitioners for a variety of conditions. Certainly in the latter two cases, the patients revealed high degrees of knowledgeability and control over their health and were able to envisage situations where they would see their doctor and when it would be more appropriate to use their practitioner. In other words the users may "use" both alternative and biomedical care but for different problems, biomedicine being regarded as particularly important for acute conditions and accidents. It also suggests that patients are not dissatisfied with biomedicine *per se* but are perhaps dissatisfied with the treatments for a specific ailment. Cant's (1997) qualitative study of patients also revealed similar "demarcated" use.[4] As patients became more educated about their chosen therapy they were more inclined to seek care without recourse to the general practitioner but there were always situations when they could envisage using biomedicine: "I'd always go to the homoeopath first if it was not life threatening, if it was causing serious discomfort or if it was acute I'd probably go to the GP.", or, "I only take antibiotics now in an emergency. I used to go to the general practitioner ten times a year, now I only go twice and that's with a gall bladder problem."

Moreover, if we focus on specific therapies as with Sawyer & Ramlow's work in America we see that patients can become educated about the benefits of, in this case chiropractic, and will then always consult these practitioners as a first health care option, treating them as primary practitioners and will not attend the biomedical clinic for certain conditions (Sawyer & Ramlow 1984). This also shows us that dissatisfaction with biomedicine is seldom total and cannot account entirely for the recourse to alternative medical practitioners (an area we shall discuss more fully in the next section) but also that we must understand the use of the alternative medicine as a process. Patients may undergo trajectories of experience that enable them in time to use the various services selectively.

Nevertheless, even if there is evidence that the lay public use the various services selectively it still appears that biomedical practitioners are uninformed about their patient's use of alternative medical services (Cant & Calnan 1991, Sharma 1992). In Cant's study[4] one respondent talked of being frightened of telling her general practitioner and other biomedical personnel that she used alternative medical services: "I didn't tell the hospital that I was taking a remedy, it felt like I was taking one system into another, but I always tell the homoeopath which orthodox drugs I am taking."

It may be, as in the case above, that the homoeopath always asked about orthodox medication, and perhaps that biomedical doctors have still not accustomed themselves to such questioning. However, it also suggests that whereas consumers may seek plural health care options, the biomedical practitioners are not necessarily aware of the extent of such usage among their patients.

The majority of users are directed to alternative medicine by recommendation from friends or family (local networks) and not via the advertisements placed by practitioners or through the media. This does not mean that consumers have no information or interest in the therapy and consume without thought. On the contrary, Sharma (1992) found that her respondents had informed themselves about the therapy and possible cures for their problem but that the actual choice of practitioner was made on the basis of advice from "significant others". Similarly, in Australia, Lloyd et al. (1993) found that after personal recommendation (64 per cent), personal assessment of practitioners after shopping around was the next most frequent means of identifying a therapist and that 78 per cent of patients had accurate and detailed knowledge of the qualifications held by their practitioners. This seems to suggest a degree of active consumerism, that patients are knowledgeable and informed, but this may be more likely for those users that do not go through personal recommendation. For example, in a recent qualitative study[4], respondents were surprised, on being questioned, that they had not made themselves more knowledgeable about their practitioner's qualifications and about how the therapy worked: "How interesting that I didn't ask (about qualifications), maybe I ought to, I suppose I trust him now."

Another did not feel the need to examine the practitioner: "No, not at all, I know a person that went to him and if it was okay for them, I knew it was okay for me. To me everything is liking the person, so I am less interested in qualifications."

It is interesting that the consumers place such trust in the practitioners at a time when the practitioners themselves are so concerned that they prove themselves to be qualified (see Ch. 3) and when the government and the medical profession have exerted strong pressure, in the name of the consumer, upon the alternative practitioners to prove themselves to be trained (see Ch. 4 and Ch. 5).

In turn, the new and satisfied users of course act as advisors to other users or they actively bring new users to the practitioner (as in the case of mothers who decide to use it for their children, particularly when concerned about the over use of antibiotics). This seemed to be a frequent pattern (Sharma 1992). Once the parent had tried the therapy for themselves they were happy to use it with their children. Women of course may not have the same success with their partners. In Cant's (1997)[4] study for instance, one respondent talked about how she had convinced all her children to use the homoeopath but could not get her husband to attend: "No, he's on a different planet, he'd say he had no time, but you need to be a sensitive type of person to go. Women think more about themselves, they are more aware of their bodies."

Overall, can we say that illness behaviour is any different among users of alternative medicine? In terms of lay referrals and the gathering of advice from local networks, it can be argued that this is merely a replication of help seeking within the biomedical sector. There seems to be some evidence that consumers of alternative medicine do gather advice about their condition and shop around, but this could be a feature of having a chronic health problem. What is certain is that the patterns of use are not static but change over time as consumers become more acquainted with the skills of the alternative medical practitioner and consequently we must understand the use of this sector as processual. For the majority of users simultaneous care from orthodox and alternative practitioners is the norm rather than the exception although there is some evidence that the consumers are knowledgeable about appropriate care and in effect choose between practitioners on the basis of their medical problem. This would seem to provide evidence of pluralism – patients actively and consciously choose from a range of practitioners and services and use these services selectively rather than simply adding to or "topping up" biomedical care.

Motivations to consume

Thus far the discussion has alluded to a number of possible individual motivations for turning to alternative medicine. However, we need to examine these reasons more carefully to assess whether they offer general explanations for the increased popularity and the rise of the new medical pluralism. At the most simplistic level the examination of the dissatisfactions with biomedicine and the attractions of alternative medicine offer some insight into this question, but as we shall see the picture is rather more complicated and is not a case of individual consumers weighing up costs and benefits in a calculated manner. The decision making process is a complex one and incorporates perceptions of the body, desire for inclusion and power in the healing process.

Let us first take the more straightforward explanations as given by the consumers. Sharma's study offers ample evidence of the costs and benefits of using alternative and orthodox medical services. We can link the use of alternative medicine to wider concerns about modern science. Specifically, it appears that many consumers are genuinely concerned about the side effects of drugs and are anxious about taking medication that seems to them to be made of artificial substances and chemicals. In contrast, the apparent harmlessness of alternative medicine and its concentration on natural products is an attraction:

> Jason had a very bad skin rash which would not clear up, and I thought it might be eczema. The doctor prescribed cortisone creams and steroids which I thought was rather drastic. We went to a homoeopath who dealt with the problem more or less. It was a relief not to have put cortisone cream and stuff like that all over his hands . . . I was always worried about having medicine in the house and I was relieved that homoeopathic medicines are non-poisonous. If you take a whole bottle full you are not going to die even though it may be labelled "belladonna" or something like that. (Sharma 1996a: 236)

Or

> I tried all the tablets the GP gave me for my migraine. I have had all kinds, Migraleve, Migril etc which I don't believe in because they have got ergotamines and I feel the side effects are too great and I am not prepared to risk it. I think it is too much. (Sharma 1996a: 237)

Of course, consumers may be under some misapprehension if they automatically equate alternative medicine with safety and the BMA has gone to great lengths to point out the potential harm that can come from consultations with alternative practitioners (BMA 1986, 1987). These include the failure of alternative practitioners to identify serious medical conditions and the side effects associated with alternative medical products (this was the basis of the campaign to ban comfrey, although in this case, as Whitelegg (1996) shows, the evidence against the herb was far from convincing).

It is also the case, as we have already seen, that consumers of alternative medicine are concerned about the effectiveness of bio-medicine and its ability to provide answers to chronic health problems (Donnelly et al. 1985, Moore et al. 1985, Furnham & Smith 1988). MacGregor & Peay (1996) showed that while users of alternative medicine were not necessarily dissatisfied with their recent visits to their biomedical practitioners, they expressed lower levels of confidence in biomedicine in general. Perhaps the most obvious reason for continuing to use alternative medicine is the experience that it is efficacious, and a number of respondents in Cant's study suggested that they had been won over to homoeopathy because they had experienced positive results: "I really had bad ovulating pain, he gave me a remedy and it worked. That was what converted me. Homoeopathy worked in five minutes, no more pain. It was so miraculous."

Another interviewee recognized that she could not prove that it was homoeopathy that had made her feel better: "The remedy worked in a very gradual way, I mean you could be getting better yourself. That's the airy fairy nature of homoeopathy."

Indeed, surveys of users have found widespread satisfaction with alternative medicine. For example, in a *Guardian* (1996) survey all except four of the 386 respondents claimed to have experienced some improvement in their condition. Maybe the continued motivation to use this sector is a pragmatic one? It is important to try and locate the foundations upon which feelings of satisfaction are based, as it is unlikely that alternative medicine is judged purely on clinical efficacy but also the extent to which consumers feel that their experiences are taken seriously and given due attention and time.

This leads us to another area of concern to consumers – the amount of time that is spent with the practitioner. All studies have revealed that consumers are drawn to consultations where they have more opportunity to discuss their problem in depth.

> They [complementary practitioners] give you more time. Obviously most of them charge you, so they would do. But most of them treat the individual symptoms as the individual's problem not just some Latinised name (Sharma 1996a: 242).

Or as a respondent in Cant's study also explained,

> I tend to get depressed and then I get fat because I eat more. The general practitioner said to go out more and use prozac. You just get a prescription but you don't get to the bottom of

why you are depressed because they haven't got the time to get to the root cause and because they have not been trained to treat you totally and wholly.

Most first consultations with alternative practitioners tend to last well over an hour (Sharma 1992, Cant & Calnan 1991) although again we must be cautious about making generalizations. Some therapists do not need to spend as long with the patient, for example the average consultation with a chiropractor lasts between 15 and 20 minutes (Cant & Sharma 1994). Perhaps in the case of chiropractic it is the pragmatic and physical relief that is important rather than the detailed discussion of a person's emotional, and spiritual well-being, as might be the case in a two-hour session with a homoeopath? Certainly, the attraction of time is not peculiar to alternative medicine and studies of the private biomedical sector have revealed this to be an important reason for choosing to pay (Calnan et al. 1993). The issue of time, however, is also a contentious one; discussions within therapy groups about the advantages and disadvantages of incorporating their practice into the National Health Service always reveal concerns that such a move would necessarily curtail the amount of time the practitioner could spend with their patients (see Ch. 6).

If we move beyond the straightforward costs and benefits to patients of biomedicine versus alternative medicine another range of explanations become available, in particular motivations that resonate with wider cultural changes. The increased availability of information and the knowledge of risks may have provided for a more reflexive and questioning consumer – an explanation that of course precedes those of costs and benefits. In Sharma's study there was evidence of interviewees who had developed greater confidence in their capacity to choose between therapies: "I make up my own mind about these things now . . . Now I feel I am in control of my life." (Sharma 1995:51).

It appears that patients also desire more control in the consultation. In longer consultations patients have the opportunity to provide more information about their complaint and take on board information provided by the practitioners (Johannessen 1996). Qualitative studies have revealed that patients respond to being treated as an equal and desire a more participative relationship with their practitioner (Hewer 1983). Such a possibility derives from the fact that most alternative medicine proposes a form of holism, which rejects the treatment of symptoms in isolation but seeks to understand them in the context of a person's total health profile (their spiritual and emotional responses as well as their experience of their social situation). Such an approach requires both an individualistic approach to treatment and the need to extract detailed information from the patient about the circumstances of their illness and their feelings about it. Consequently, the patient is given the position of "expert", having valuable knowledge about themselves and this is clearly enjoyed. As one respondent in Sharma's study revealed: "When I saw her I thought she is of my intelligence, she treats me as an equal." (Sharma 1995:51).

Similarly in Cant's[4] study, the positive aspects of mutuality again were expressed: "He takes my opinion more seriously, I have more time and it is more two way definitely, but obviously he makes the decision about the remedy." Or, "I really connect with him, I have a relationship with him, I feel comfortable and trust the person. He's not just your clinician, he's caring."

Many of the respondents in this study spoke about their practitioner as being a friend or confidante as much as a practitioner. As one woman said: "He's the third most important man in my life after my husband and son."

In many of the cases this made the relationship a rather ambiguous one, for after all the practitioner is not usually a friend, although the patient may feel that they have connected with him/her in the consultation room and experience feelings of closeness. The following extract from Cant's study is revealing,

> I unburden myself and he listens . . . I still go now that I am well and talk to him about any old thing. But he has suggested that I do not see him for a while. I feel really quite sorry, my husband is away a lot and I enjoyed unburdening myself.

Indeed one respondent talked of how she had expected the homoeopath to check up on her on an occasion when she had been admitted to hospital and "I felt really upset when he did not ring – I felt let down really."

Thus, a more mutual and sharing relationship also brings ambiguities, ones that have to be dealt with carefully. One homoeopath told how she had two phones in her home, one number for her personal friends and one for her patients, that she could leave on the answer machine and monitor if patients were becoming too intrusive (Cant 1997)[4]. The professional associations that represent practitioners have also had to reflect upon this problem and have drawn up clear codes of conduct so that any claims of harassment or misunderstanding made by patients can be dealt with in a clear manner.

Although all the respondents that were questioned in Cant's study felt that they had a role to play in the consultation, the majority were not at all informed about the medication that they had been prescribed or indeed about homoeopathy in general; indeed only one respondent said that they had read up about the remedy that they had been given: "I never know which remedy I have been given. I never know what the remedy is – I did read and go to lectures, I got hooked really, but he (the homoeopath) discouraged me and told me to think that it is all magic".

Such a description of the consultation suggests a number of possible interpretations. Perhaps there is a level where patients do not wish to exercise knowledgeability and consumerism, just as in the private biomedical sector where the patients do not make the choice of consultant (Calnan et al. 1993). It may also be the case that practitioners only want to encourage a degree of participation, partly no doubt to maintain their own distance and boundaries of expertise (see Cant & Sharma 1996b, 1996d). Or perhaps there is a concern to protect the patient; for example, in homoeopathy there is often a reluctance to tell patients about the chosen remedy, which is linked to a whole range of social and emotional traits (e.g. tearful, greedy, etc.) because the practitioners are concerned that the patient may read the descriptions and make assumptions about how the practitioner viewed their personality. Overall, however, patients talked of feeling that they were participating in the medical encounter. According to Taylor (1984) this shift links more to changes in the political rather than medical culture and demands for the democratization of decision-making. Certainly, this view would link in with Giddens's (1990) discussion of the growing disillusionment with the expert, and processes of re-skilling by the lay populace.

This idea also resonates with an explanation offered by medical anthropologists that suggests alternative medicine offers more meaning to the patients and allows them to link their illness to wider cultural, personal and social frameworks. We know that the lay public have a wide range of frameworks that they use to make sense of illness episodes and that they use illness episodes to re-interpret their own biographies. These frameworks – such as a previous experience or the health of other family members – are not generally drawn upon by the biomedical doctor. In contrast, alternative medical practitioners usually spend a long time questioning the patients about their family, their lifestyle and environment (indeed questions can be so probing and seemingly irrelevant that new patients can feel perturbed about their relevance). Helman puts great emphasis on the sense making potential of alternative medicine, especially that which it gives to suffering:

> Many patients have an unfulfilled sense of wanting to be connected once again, to some wider context, to locate their suffering in a wider framework – even to somehow contain themselves within the many cycles of nature ... Complementary practitioners often help people make sense of their situation in a more meaningful way than does medicine, often utilising more traditional modes of dealing with misfortune ... many of them utilise traditional cultural beliefs in order to explain to the patient why they have been affected by that particular illness at that particular time. (Helman 1992:12)

Certainly there seems to be some evidence that patients feel that alternative medicine does help them make sense of their situation even if it is by simply linking their health problems to those of their family. As one respondent in Sharma's study outlined,

> I had to do a massive questionnaire about my family background. No-one had ever asked me to do this before. I had to ring my mother and go back to bronchial asthma in my family before the turn of the century ... all this seems to come together and it was *my* body and *my* temperament. (Sharma 1996a:243)

Thus, alternative medicine may offer new ways of looking at health and illness that move beyond reductionist accounts and allow for more varied and plural understandings that converge with those held by the patient. Johannessen (1996) argues that the individualized treatment bestows meaning to the patient and allows them to create order in a situation of personal chaos, created by the illness episode. The explanations offered by the alternative practitioner purport to be and are experienced by the patient as "tailor made" to their own biography and experiences and can in turn engender changes to the person's perception of their health and social situation. Such a stance clearly also allows the patients the opportunity to develop and extend their pluralistic understandings of their bodies and bodily suffering and to construct multiple possibilities for comprehending the relationship between their body, self and social context (Busby 1996).

It is also possible that the motivations to use alternative medicine may stem from changes to attitudes held about the body, although it is difficult to establish whether it is ideas about the body that motivate use or whether consumers alter their perception of their body as a consequence of visiting an alternative therapist. Certainly, at a time when the body has come to be seen as a "project" (Giddens 1991, Shilling 1993), it is not hard to see the attraction of therapeutic practice that places great emphasis on a holistic approach to health care and which makes links between physical complaints and the emotional and spiritual levels of a person and indeed offers hope that good health can be achieved and maintained. According to Coward, alternative medicine is premised on very different ideas about the body and assumes that perfect health is an achievable aim. "The body has a whole new centrality as a place of work and transformation." (Coward 1989: 194).

The long term users of homoeopathy in Cant's study[4] had found that they were more aware of their bodies and tended to monitor physical changes more closely, especially recognizing that these may be a sign that they were emotionally unwell. Such body monitoring is often encouraged by the therapists who sometimes ask their patients to keep a diary of how they are feeling and to chart any bodily changes they experience. Respondents felt they had altered in their perceptions of themselves:

> It has done something to me – what am I trying to say, my body tells me what is happening all the time. My body leads me now ... if the psoriasis starts I know now that I am emotionally stressed ... I make the connection between emotional and

physical signs. I don't check my body all the time but I do monitor it.

Another interviewee said:

Maybe you become a bit of a hypochondriac. I think everything is now relevant. I think about my whole body and how it might be connected. The body constantly surprises you when you monitor it.

Others talked about how they had become more obsessed with their good health and made sure that they did all possible to ensure that a state of such "good health" was maintained: "I am more aware of my body, its strengths and weaknesses. I go to the homoeopath because I am worried about the winter and I go for a boost . . . my health rules my life really."

These extracts concur with Lloyd et al.'s (1993) findings that users were concerned about having a healthy lifestyle but this also places responsibility upon the individual to ensure they monitor and judge all physical, mental and spiritual changes that they experience. There was evidence in many of the interviews (Cant 1997)[4] that using homoeopathy had provided the interviewees with a broader understanding of their bodies, their health and a recognition of their obligations if they wished to achieve perfect wellbeing: "I've learnt to exercise more and to eat differently and I am aware that everything is connected." Or, "Homoeopathy touches your whole life and you understand yourself, I do not know how I lived without it."

Such commentary can explain the continued use of alternative therapies and also illustrates the connection between alternative medical practice and "healthism" (Crawford 1980) – the desire to retain and maintain perfectibility in health and put much of the emphasis upon the individual. This emphasis can of course be interpreted as empowering, offering individuals the opportunity to know themselves (Busby 1996) or as disciplining, deflecting the responsibility away from society and operating as a surveillance function (Braathen 1996). Crawford (1980) would use the latter interpretation, arguing that alternative medicine does not empower the individual as this would require effective social and political analysis of the causes of ill health. Certainly alternative medicine seems to demedicalize personal health by encouraging the individual to be less dependant on biomedicine but paradoxically it remedicalizes life, bringing all areas of a person's emotional and spiritual life under scrutiny (Lowenberg & Davis 1994).

Conclusion

Despite the cost-disincentives of using alternative medicine we have seen a significant and progressive increase in the use of alternative practitioners across the Western world. How can such a situation be explained and what do we learn when we examine lay views and experiences of the alternative medical sector? There certainly seems to be some evidence that alternative medicine has become popular because of the discontent felt towards biomedicine, although these dissatisfactions seem to be fairly specific (especially side-effects of drugs) as we are not seeing a major shift away from biomedicine itself. This is not at all surprising when we consider the advantages of biomedicine rather than its faults: it is important not to deny the effectiveness of biomedicine in the relief of many areas of illness (Kelly & Field 1994). Indeed many consumers recognize the clinical effectiveness of biomedicine but prefer to seek care that is less invasive and more natural. It is unlikely that consumers were ever fully convinced by the claims of biomedicine but perhaps the preparedness to use alternative medicine does signify greater knowledge on the part of the patients and that they may hold increasingly contradictory ideas about biomedicine, recognizing the advantages but not necessarily ready to risk the consequences of use in every situation. Despite concerns about the simultaneous use of biomedical and alternative medical services, there is evidence that with increased usage and faith in alternative medicine, consumers are increasingly sophisticated in their choice of health care, seeing each sector as having its appropriate areas of competence. Nevertheless, the rise in the use of alternative medicine does coincide with the ever increasing use of biomedical services and questions have to be asked about the rising expectations and demands held by the consumer. Whereas the variety of usage patterns means that it is important that we recognize that the use of the alternative medical sector is a complex question, it does appear that we are seeing a pluralistic and "complementary" system of health care developing. However, the continuing reluctance on the part of the patient to tell their general practitioner that they use these services may mean this plural use of services continues to be a clandestine activity.

Hopefully we have shown that it is difficult to unpack the motivations to use alternative medicine. This is partly the product of methodological problems: you have to ask users to talk about their experiences retrospectively and their accounts may be coloured by their subsequent experience of a particular therapy. For example, while it is widely held by users of alternative medicine that the relationship with the orthodox doctor is impersonal and mechanistic, did they only appreciate this after visiting an alternative practitioner? Consequently, we may need to comprehend the rise of the plural use of medical services as a process and introduce the idea of a trajectory into our analysis, recognizing that experiences will vary from user to user. Some may consult because they hold particular health ideologies, require a different relationship with their practitioner, are concerned about the safety of biomedicine or find that alternative medicine offers them multiple ways of understanding their bodies, bodily suffering and making sense of their illness in relation to their own biography and social and cultural context. Others may be more pragmatic, desiring the relief of a particular symptom. We must also learn another lesson from this study and be wary of treating alternative medicine and its attractions as a whole. In other words, therapy specific analysis is essential as is work that follows patients through their experiences of alternative medicine and acknowledges their attempts to use the consultation as a means of making sense of their own illness and identity.

There are also problems when we wish to assess data that shows that users have healthier lifestyles (Lloyd et al. 1993), are more appreciative of exercise and healthy eating or may seem to be very reflexive about their bodies. Considering that many alternative medical practitioners view their practice as educative, we have difficulty in showing at what point these ideas and views became more important to the user.

The explanations that are offered by the users of alternative medicine do seem to resonate with some of the themes highlighted by Giddens (1990) in his description of late modernity, namely risk, and the desire for participation and individual attention. More than this, the processes of help seeking in this sector link into Giddens' discussion of trust. Here Giddens argues that the lay public will always be dependent upon experts to translate knowledge for them, and although they may re-skill and attempt to re-appropriate knowledge, the choice of alternatives will also require a "leap in faith". What is striking in Cant's (1997)[4] work is this display of trust, although we cannot be certain how long this may last. Of course, the users tend to depend on personal recommendation and so are confident that the practitioner has been "tried and tested" but nevertheless there was a disinterest in the credentials and standing of the therapists.

It is possible for us to make some tentative statements about the significance of the increased popularity of alternative medicine and this new medical pluralism. At one level, if we take on board the medicalizing impact of alternative medicine we might argue that alternative medical practice perpetuates many of the features of biomedicine. Neither seek to improve the social conditions in which people live and both place a degree of responsibility upon the individual. Although alternative medicine may appear to be novel, it may simply be an extension of biomedical concerns? At the same time the re-emergence of alternative modes of thought and practices pertaining to health and illness may lead to a re-negotiation of the social contract of health, which could have implications for the power and hegemony of biomedicine. The greater scepticism towards biomedicine among users is testimony to this, and if the use of alternative medicine continues to increase we may see a displacing of the doctor's position of authority. The users of alternative medicine appreciate the equality that they feel in their dealings with their practitioner, even if this can produce ambiguities. As patients become more valued as experts in the healing process, providing information that is otherwise inaccessible to the practitioner, it is possible that we may see medicine becoming more patient centred. Biomedicine has recognized this attraction (BMA 1986) and doctors may become more open to such a relationship themselves. These are all areas that need to be studied more closely but imply that pluralism can be conservative as well as radical.

By deciding to use alternative medicine it appears that the patient may have become a consumer. Clearly, the expansion of the alternative medical sector produces a wider market of services from which a person can choose and while this continues to be concentrated in the private sector it is likely that the advice of the general practitioner will not be as important as the consumer's own decision. Paying for the services also places the consumer in a similar position to the patient of bedside medicine (Jewson 1976), practitioners are dependant upon the patronage of their users for their livelihood and consequently the power of the consumer is greater. Here we see how pluralism might be termed *new* – because where the lay public have been shown to always hold conflicting, complex and different ideas about health and illness, the use of alternative medicine requires the user to move from a dependent position as patient to an active one as consumer.

While we need to examine the use of alternative medicine therapy by therapy to gain real insight into the nature of demand, the expansion of a very broad range of approaches that call themselves "therapies" means that we can make a general observation about what constitutes health care and health related behaviour. What is the significance of the expansion in use of beauty therapies, hairdresser salons called "hair and health" and a range of therapies that concentrate on exercise and deportment? Perhaps we can no longer define health using biomedical and physical definitions. Rather, "good health" should be seen as the product of spiritual, emotional and physical wellbeing and this in turn must blur the boundaries between what have been understood as medical, recreational and aesthetic techniques of the body.

Sociologists may argue about the significance of the new medical pluralism but what is certain is that it is widespread, with figures suggesting that about a third of adults have used alternative medicine at some time. As such, this is not a fringe activity and now represents a variation of normal illness behaviour. However, there does seem to be evidence that there are still gender and class divisions in usage patterns, ones that may shift if alternative medicine is made freely available within state funded health care. However, at the current time in Britain at least, the use of alternative medicine is not evenly distributed, but is concentrated in areas where practitioners are situated and to a small number of therapies. Pluralism is consequently constrained by the supply of practitioners. Nevertheless, they too seem to be increasing in number and professionalism and it is to their story that we now turn.

Notes

1. To talk of lay health beliefs, the lay perspective and the lay public should be recognized as a shorthand description and is not intended to convey any sense that the lay populace is homogeneous or indeed fixed. On the contrary, the lay public should be recognized as heterogeneous, multi-vocal, and as holding complex and changing views and attitudes.
2. Beliefs and attitudes are of course always expressed in a situational context and can vary accordingly. Consequently it is hard to capture these views, to establish stability in expressed opinion, or show how people's beliefs may have shifted.
3. *WHICH?* is a publication of a consumer association in Britain.
4. The data comes from a recently completed study of 20 consumers of homoeopathy, part of a doctoral programme of research.

CHAPTER 3

From "alternative" to "complementary": revival and transformation

The laws of supply and demand require that the accelerated con-sumption of alternative medicine be matched by increased provision of therapies and practitioners. The expansion of the alternative medical services was characterized by the revival of therapies that had previously been popular and the arrival of therapies from abroad. In this chapter we tell the story of the pluralization of the health services[1] from the perspective of the alternative therapy groups themselves, with our major focus being upon non-medically qualified practitioners who practice in Britain.[2] (The operation of "common law"[3] in the United Kingdom provides for legal but un-regulated practice of alternative medicine and consequently our discussion may be peculiar to this country, the absence of extensive comparative data preventing us from making wider generaliza-tions.) The rapid growth of the alternative medical services in the 1980s provoked critical interest from the consumers, but also from governments and, of course, from the medical profession, so much so that the alternative therapists could not simply practice but had to attend to questions of their own legitimacy, organization and train-ing and their place in the health service.

There is not a single narrative to this British story, rather the multiple histories and expectations of the various therapy groups and the differing perceptions of their role in the health care market provide for a number of possible end points. While this chapter will chart the general changes made by the alternative medical groups, we do not assume that there are a sequence of stages on a con-tinuum that ranges from unorganized and illegitimate at one end of

51

the spectrum to coherent and approved at the other, through which all groups must move.

In the first place, the complexity of the alternative medical market means that all therapy communities do not have the same goals. For example, it is estimated that there are over 160 therapies currently available in the United Kingdom (HMSO 1987), differing in the way that they are organized and what they purport to treat. Nevertheless, it is possible to produce typologies to demarcate alternative medicine (see Ch. 1 for one such model). Pietroni's (1992) typology is particularly relevant to this chapter as he divides the alternative medical field into four types based on their knowledge claims, a categorization that was also adopted by the medical profession in Britain. "Complete" systems of medicine refer to those therapies that claim to offer a whole system of medicine. In this, Petrioni included homoeopathy, herbal medicine, acupuncture, osteopathy and chiropractic. It is interesting to note that these therapies are also those that are most commonly used and also have the longest training programmes. The label of "complete" has some problems as it should not be equated with the idea that the therapies make claims to treat all medical complaints – this is patently not the case with modern chiropractic for example and its concentration on lower back problems (see Ch. 5 for more details). The next two categories are similar in the sense that they generally require less formal teaching but differ in terms of the claims they make for their therapy – here Petrioni makes a distinction between "diagnostic" (e.g. iridology) and "therapeutic" (e.g. reflexology) modalities. Finally, "self help" approaches, such as meditation and relaxation, often do not require the presence of a practitioner.

It is, of course, possible for us to demarcate the therapies in many other ways, for example in terms of how the various groups see their role in the health service and in particular their relationship with biomedicine. More radical therapies may perceive themselves to be entirely "alternative", any collaboration with biomedicine being anathema to their practice and ideological underpinnings. Others may view themselves as equal partners in the health care market – a "complementary" relationship, or may view their practice as subordinate or supplementary to biomedical practice. Still others see themselves as an educative presence, as in the case of the

Alexander Technique. Moreover, these categorizations are never fixed.

Secondly, in this chapter the major focus is upon the "official" representatives and representations of the therapy groups. However, this is only one narrative, the public representation if you like, which coexists alongside many different representations and understandings of how each therapy should be practised and presented. For example, many individual therapists do not choose to belong to their official professional associations.[4] Such practitioners usually practice more than one therapy (Sharma 1992), although may designate one approach as their main profession, and are likely not to belong to associations or participate in discussions pertaining to their subsidiary practice either. They often practice in highly individualistic ways (Johannessen 1996). We will be drawing out examples of how the therapy groups have produced an "official" line about the content of education and the correct place of their therapy, but internally the professional groups are not necessarily in agreement with such a portrayal and their professional journals contain much discussion and argument about these issues (see Sharma 1996). The increasing number of practitioners has further complicated matters, potentially multiplying the divergent views about each therapy. Estimates (although these are difficult to corroborate) suggest that the increase in the number of practitioners is exponential. In the United Kingdom, extrapolations from survey material collected in 1981 (see Fulder (1988) for data and estimates by Sharma (1992)), produced a figure of 26,483 therapists. This figure is clearly outdated and, in 1997, one pan-professional body alone claimed to represent 60,000 therapists.[5] In the United States, one study (Cooper & Stoflet 1996) has shown that the number of chiropractors trebled between 1970 and 1990 and has projected that the per capita supply of alternative medical clinicians will increase by a further 88 per cent by 2010. Consequently, the public narrative is always a contentious one.

Thirdly, and as a caveat to this chapter, we want to argue that any sociological study of alternative medical groups and the changes they undergo must be wary of the desire to make comparisons with the established medical profession. Biomedicine, throughout the world, has established itself as a highly trained, internally regulated and "professional" occupation. Sociologists have expended enormous effort in the description and interpretation of the occupational project of biomedicine and have isolated key traits of professional groups (e.g. Greenwood 1957), describing those groups that do not meet the criteria as in some way occupationally inferior, but as having the potential to aspire to such heady heights with the right amount of commitment and endeavour. This mode of analysis has been discredited (Freidson 1970) but many writers (e.g. Wardwell 1992) still assume an inevitability to the changes expected of, or available to, alternative medical groups and the correct/proper or valid forms of occupational development. We wish to move beyond such a judgemental reading. In particular, the dominance of biomedicine often blinkers us to alternative organizational forms, coaxes us to look for similarities to that particular orthodox format and prevents us from recognizing that other occupational groups can be proactive in their choice of occupational route, not merely acquiescent to the demands of a more powerful competitor.

This is not to say that the biomedical profession is immaterial. As we shall see in the next chapter, the medical profession is, on the contrary, a powerful player and it is unlikely that the alternative medical practitioners would have been able to ignore the demands of this group or fail to take note of the strategies that medicine took to promote its own interests. However, as sociologists we must not judge the status of alternative medicine against this archetypal example of a profession. Historically the sociology of alternative medicine has tended to fall into this trap and view alternative medical groups in some way as inadequate or limited (Wardwell 1994).[6] It is possible to describe the organizational changes undertaken by the therapy groups without resorting to a discussion of their relative standing or by assuming that alterations have been accepted in a non reflective and unconscious manner.

This is important because we know that sociology does feed back its findings and ideas into the environment that it studies – what Giddens (1990) referred to as the "double hermeneutic", the potential of academic studies to not simply describe social processes but in some part constitute them. Already our own work has been used by one complementary group in the United Kingdom as evidence that they are involved in scientific research (see BMA 1993). Therefore, to describe alternative medical groups as in some way marginal, or to use other such value laden concepts, in turn defines the terrain of the health care market and can, as Coulter (1991) argues, serve to actually reinforce medical hegemony.

Bearing in mind the complexity of the field and the problems of comparison, we will attempt to make some general observations about what has happened within alternative medicine in the last thirty years in Britain and will argue that many of the groups have engaged in significant changes to the way that they train, practice and perceive their role in the health service (the "official" discourse) and, moreover, that this has entailed some "convergence" with biomedicine (hence the title of this chapter).

The revival of "alternative" medicine

At one level, to talk of the revival of alternative medicine is to overlook the fact that many therapies have maintained a constant place in the overall medical provision in most societies. In some countries there has always been a vibrant alternative to biomedicine, especially where the services are difficult or expensive to obtain (Baer 1984a). However, it is possible to show that in many places alternative medicine was popular but then experienced a period of decline to be followed by a revival in the 1970s, which included the popularization of indigenous therapies and the arrival of therapies from abroad. For example, across Europe there is evidence that in spite of different levels of support from the various governments and medical professions, many therapies became more popular (e.g. Vaskilampi's (1993) work in Finland), although there are differences in the types of therapies that have become more favoured. For example, in Denmark alternative therapies became more popular from the 1970s (Staugård 1993) but this was especially the case for reflexology. In contrast, in Iceland (Haraldsson 1993) and Holland (Fisher & Ward 1994) there has been an exponential increase in the usage of spiritual healers, whereas in France acupuncture and homoeopathy have become very popular (Traverso 1993). The revival of alternative medicine in Australia (Willis 1989) and the USA (Sale 1995) parallels developments in Europe although there is much evidence that in the United States therapies such as chiropractic, osteopathy and naturopathy (Baer 1992) maintained a strong presence throughout the century but experienced further rejuvenation in the 1970s. There are also clear differences across Europe when the training and academic background of the practitioner is examined. In countries with more restrictive legal systems (see Ch. 5 for more details), such as Belgium and France, the expansion of therapies has been confined to doctors or other recognized and medically orientated professionals such as physiotherapists.

Following Weber (1968), it is possible to describe the 1970s revival of many therapies as practised by non-medically qualified practitioners as charismatic,[7] (obviously this did not apply to the more established therapies – their charismatic phases occurring in the 1890s in the case of chiropractic and osteopathy). The proponents were treated as leaders and had extraordinary qualities that inspired enthusiasm in their followers. Fulder (1996) suggests that charismatic teaching was responsible for the arrival of acupuncture in the West and it is possible to identify key individuals in the revival of complementary medicine in the United Kingdom who taught in an unstructured way, bestowing their insight to dedicated followers who came from all walks of life and did not require any specific credentials beyond enthusiasm.

The charismatic nature of the revival of non-medically qualified homoeopathy in the United Kingdom stands as a case in point. Although homoeopathy was founded as a specific medical treatment in the late eighteenth century in Germany, and quickly became popular with medical doctors in Britain, the practice went into decline after the Second World War despite the support of the royal family. Moreover, homoeopathy, as practised by the medical establishment took on a particular complexion, homoeopathic remedies being used in conjunction with allopathic medicine (Nicholls 1988, Cant & Sharma 1994, 1996d). However, during the 1970s homoeopathy took on a new direction, promoted by two non-medically qualified practitioners, Da Monte and Maughan, who were also Druids.[8] Each proponent independently incorporated homoeopathic healing practices into their Druidic philosophy and attracted a dedicated following from their students. As one of the homoeopaths we interviewed recounted:

> each had a small group of students who were attracted by affinity. And you did not just get homoeopathy but a whole point of view. You just knew that you were getting a huge well of knowl-

edge just by attending his classes. He taught us about the meaning of life and many of us became Druids.

Or

> Well, it was different then, not so structured. We learned from a man who was really an esoteric philosopher . . . and he used radionics and pendulums . . . we had all been treated by him and wanted to learn more.

There was no structure to the teaching or a curriculum, rather these two men would talk about homoeopathy alongside other bodies of knowledge that were far removed from the teachings of medical homoeopathy. There was a great emphasis upon the spirituality of homoeopathy, the vital force and constitutional/individualized prescribing[9] and the students felt they had discovered something that would revolutionize medical practice:

> We wanted to spread this to people because we saw [homoeopathy] having inestimable value and wanted to get people out of the allopathic straitjacket. So the motivating force was love . . . we were very euphoric, shall I say about homoeopathy and idealistic. I wanted to shout from the rooftops. Homoeopathy was a vehicle for spiritual change and growth.

The homoeopathy that was taught was very different to that practised by medically qualified doctors in Britain, who had taken short, structured and examinable courses at the Faculty of Homoeopathy. Medical homoeopaths were using homoeopathic remedies alongside allopathic medicine and were more likely to use "pathological" prescribing, where a remedy is chosen on the basis of the disease category from which the patient suffers rather than the patient's individual constitution. Non-medically qualified homoeopathy thus re-emerged as a highly individualistic movement and, furthermore, the teachings placed great emphasis upon an interactive and non-hierarchical relationship with the patient. There was far more concern about the spread of homoeopathic ideals than about the accreditation of homoeopathic knowledge and professional training. There were no stipulations about who could study as it was felt that the best way of expanding the popularity of the approach was to train as many people as possible. Therefore, in this example, we can see that the therapy was both revived and re-interpreted.

In contrast, chiropractic has had a longer history of non-medical practice but has also experienced varied reactions on being exported across the world. Emerging in the United States in 1895, the technique was taken to Britain and elsewhere in the 1920s. In spite of widespread hostility from the medical profession, chiropractic retained constant, if low, public support especially in the United States (Coburn & Biggs 1986) and consequently the establishment of training colleges occurred in the 1960s, for example in Canada (Biggs 1992) and Britain (Cant & Sharma 1994) before the great expansion in popular support in the late 1970s and 1980s. In the United Kingdom, initial popularity was curtailed by the establishment of the National Health Service but there is evidence that in the late 1970s new charismatic revivals of chiropractic (e.g. McTimoney Chiropractic) led to the emergence of different versions of the practice, taught by committed individuals to willing students who had a range of backgrounds and qualifications (see Cant 1996 and Ch. 5). Other therapies, of course, first became popular in the late 1970s. For example, reflexology gained a foothold in the United Kingdom, although it did not became as popular as in Denmark, as converts to the therapy learned the techniques abroad and brought them back home.

In very general terms the non-medical revival of these therapies, certainly in the United Kingdom, was marked by radicalism, the therapists often seeing themselves and their knowledge as separate from biomedicine, with different ideas about disease causation and appropriate forms of training and treatment. A logical extension of such a view was that the intervention of biomedicine was often seen as iatrogenic, the treatments producing side effects and dependency upon the medical regime and reducing self healing properties in the individual. Some therapists often made very grand claims for their own form of health care and tended to practice in isolation from biomedicine, even though they clearly shared the same patients. A new medical pluralism emerged at this time in the sense that there were many different systems available but the approaches were not recognized or funded by the state, were not integrated with biomedicine (indeed there was often hostility between the two groups – see Ch. 6) and they practised and trained very differently. Evidence from other countries suggest a similar generalization can be made. For example, Steffen's (1993) work about spiritual healing in Denmark depicts the revival of the therapy as culturally challenging, the approach being strongly opposed to that offered by biomedicine. Similarly, in France, Traverso (1993) suggests that in the revival of homoeopathy and acupuncture the emphasis was upon critique.

In the remainder of this chapter we show that this revival, occurring in the 1970s and 1980s, was not the end of the story. On the contrary, while there are therapists who continue to work radically and at the fringe of the medical market place (Traverso 1993, Cant & Sharma 1996c), there is substantial evidence to show that many therapists since the 1980s have collectively worked to alter the way that they train, practice and portray their therapy particularly as pressures from the state, consumers and medical profession increased.

A brief comment on the social context: the influence of key players

From the mid 1980s the revival of non-medically qualified alternative medicine could not go unnoticed and pressures increased from the other key players to alter the practices of alternative medicine. This was matched, however, by an internal recognition by the alternative practitioners themselves of the need to establish boundaries between the qualified practitioner and the lay person. (This became increasingly pertinent with the raised interest from the general public especially in homoeopathy and aromatherapy. This had led to the publication of many books about the therapies and "dabbling" by patients, indeed many therapists first became interested themselves through such experimentation – see Cant & Sharma (1994) for more details about how homoeopathic knowledge "leaked" out to the general public.) Professional practitioners became aware of the need to organize internally and to make alterations to the codification and transmission of their knowledge.

First, *governments*, as we shall explore in more detail in Chapter 5, have taken more interest in alternative medicine of recent years. This has been most apparent in the state registration of certain therapies (in the United States of America, Australia and many European countries) but with attendant demands that the various therapies prove themselves to be united and well trained – as the British Government put it – "get your act together" (HMSO 1987). The British Government has also become more interested in the educational development of therapy groups in line with their key policy of establishing National Vocational Qualifications (NVQS) as a means of developing a competent workforce and this has given rise to a project to establish National Occupational Standards for alternative medicine. Secondly, in Europe, alternative medical therapists were thrown into a panic about the prospect of a common European market and the potential demands from the *European Union* regarding the harmonization of training standards and knowledge claims across the community. The operation of Napoleonic law in some European countries restricts much complementary medical practice to biomedical doctors. As one lay homoeopath in Britain stated:

> We have been able to blossom freely here with common law . . . but it's not like that in other countries, the doctors are very powerful and they have been pressurizing the EU to outlaw non-doctors . . . so we need to harmonize our standards.

In 1997, following the Lannoye Report on unconventional medicine for the European Union,[10] the European Parliament made a number of recommendations that were important for the expansion of alternative medicine. In particular, while it is acknowledged that patients should have the "broadest possible choice of therapy" (p. 73), the European Parliament has also called for assurances that all therapists be safe, effective and qualified.

Thirdly, and as further explored in Chapter 4, the influence of the dominant *medical profession* in the occupational development of allied groups has been extensive (Donnison 1977, Larkin 1983, Willis 1989, Witz 1992). In Britain, the BMA's reaction to alternative medicine had been traditionally unfavourable. This was most clearly exhibited in the 1986 BMA report which attempted to discredit the health "alternatives" as phoney and pseudo scientific (BMA 1986). The latest BMA report (1993) is however more favourable and refers to non-biomedicine as "complementary". The shift in label from "alternative" to "complementary" signifies an acceptance that the approaches are no longer antithetic but rather "can work alongside and in conjunction with biomedical treatment" (BMA 1993:6).

Moreover, the BMA has become less interested in whether the therapies work and instead is concerned that they and their patients can be confident of the therapists' professional competence. This rather suggests then that the concern is with the trustworthiness and safety of the practitioners rather than the efficacy of their knowledge. The medical profession has certainly continued to demand that the knowledge of therapists be subject to scientific scrutiny, transmitted through proper courses, contain medical science and that biomedical practitioners should retain responsibility for the patient.

Finally, *consumer* associations[11] (e.g. ACHC 1988) have called for better training and the standardization of curricula and skills. The importance of the user for the legitimacy of occupational groups (Willis 1989) has been illustrated as practitioners have recognized the need to orient themselves to the market and make their knowledge more "acceptable" to the lay public. In the United Kingdom this concern was expressed by homoeopaths, as MacEoin (1993) states,

> The philosophy according to which a homoeopath practices must have significance to the patient . . . it may be surmised that the majority of lay homoeopaths in this country have some form of religious or esoteric commitment . . . it is hard to find lay homoeopaths who do not subscribe to New Age ideals of some kind . . . [while] this esotericism seems to have been much diluted by a broader rationalist trend . . . what worries me is the possibility that this leaning towards metaphysics instead of rational, empirically based medical practice may retard the process of broad political and scientific acceptance of homoeopathy for decades, if not indefinitely . . . Patients may feel concerned to hear of practitioners relying on intuition . . . and there are real grounds for supposing homoeopathy might as a result become ghettoised and restricted (MacEoin 1993:110–112).

All change: the transformation of content and practice

The revitalization of alternative medicine was at first often characterized by energies directed to the spread of the therapy rather than the stringent formulation of syllabi, credentials and registers of competent practitioners. Practitioners believed that their approach to health was antithetical to that offered by biomedicine (notably that the patient would be given more time, the consultation individualized and holistic). Yet the late 1980s were witness to far reaching changes at both the levels of organization and ideology, which have transformed the "official" content and practice of alternative medicine. In particular, there have been conscious attempts to alter the way that alternative medical knowledge is codified, transmitted and described and to ensure that it is demarcated from other knowledges that may be seen as illegitimate. These changes can be grouped into four major types: codification and accreditation; the tempering of knowledge claims; alignment to "science"; and the creation of boundaries around who can acquire and apply the knowledge.

Codification and accreditation

After a short period of training by charismatic leaders who paid little attention to ideas of the curricula or qualifications, the establishment of formalized colleges occurred. Of course the timing of the creation of the colleges varies by country and depends where the therapy first became popular. In Canada, for example, colleges of chiropractic emerged in the 1960s (Biggs 1992), whereas in the United Kingdom the shift from apprenticeship and unstructured teaching to a more formalized programme tended to happen later in the late 1970s and 1980s (although there are some exceptions to such a generalization – a College of Chiropractic was established in 1965, but it is true to say that concerted efforts at accreditation and particularly degree status occurred much later). Elsewhere, similar developments were also witnessed; the first colleges of naturopathy emerged in the United States (Baer 1992) and Canada (Gort and Coburn 1988) in 1978.

These developments not only marked the formalization of teaching but were also accompanied by the exponential growth in students. Baer shows that within ten years (by 1988) of the first college of naturopathy opening in the United States of America, at least 130 students were being trained a year compared to the original three students. In the UK, if we take just two of the 14 professional associations that represent reflexology, we see an exponential growth. For example, the Bayley School (albeit one of the largest) estimated in 1994 that it had trained over 3,000 reflexologists and had a membership of 374.[12] The Association of Reflexologists had 480 full members and 1,560 members overall in 1994 and suggested that 20 new members joined every week. This is a phenomenal growth when we consider that in 1984, when the Association was inaugurated, there were just ten members.

Similarly, the 1980s saw the rapid multiplication of colleges within the therapy groups. During this time, in the United States of America, another nine colleges of naturopathy emerged and in Britain, although the scale varied by therapy, there was also a significant increase in the number of colleges. For instance, within chiropractic three separate colleges had emerged by the end of the 1980s, in homoeopathy there were 20 by the early 1990s and in reflexology, at the time of writing, there were over 100 schools that had been established with no evidence that the expansion had run its course.

The "pluralization" of colleges has not simply altered *where* training takes place but has had implications for the content of the curricula and the qualifications awarded. Many therapies now have at least four years of training in addition to supervised clinical practice and increasingly there have been moves to link the courses to nationally approved credentials. For those therapies with longer programmes there have been investigations into the possibility of degree accreditation (although it is not confined to these programmes, for example, the aromatherapists are investigating the possibility of validation. See Baker 1997). At the time of writing it was possible, in the United Kingdom, to read for degrees in chiropractic, osteopathy, homoeopathy and herbalism. Aside from degree status, all colleges that we have come across have made stringent attempts to identify the necessary prerequisites for a competent practitioner and to produce a core curriculum that covers these requirements. Naturally the knowledge base of the various therapies has not become conterminous with the core curriculum, but there have been serious attempts to codify knowledge so that it can be passed on in a structured way. The retention of the principle that patients be seen as individuals now sits alongside the systematic teaching of the core curricula. Overall, the last decade has seen a significant shift from the *ad hoc* learning of skills, often on an apprenticeship basis, to the highly formalized and standardized training offered in colleges. It has also seen changes to the entry requirements to colleges, from enthusiasm and commitment to nationally recognized qualifications.

Latterly, the accreditation and standardization of the training has transcended individual colleges and has been organized by professional associations whose education committees have been concerned to publish and insist on set guidelines for education, so that standards are comparable across colleges and throughout individual countries. These associations have tended to "borrow" their organizational structure from the biomedical profession and have included an elected council, codes of ethics, a register for the practitioners, and committees to deal with education and research. The associations are generally small organizations with few, if any, paid staff. They usually produce a newsletter and journal, but in practice direct much of their attention towards the stipulation of the prerequisites of a core curriculum. They have gained status and attention from the various colleges partly because they play an important role in the representation of therapists and will only recommend courses to potential students that meet their educational criteria. As one of the directors of a reflexology association stated, the establishment of their professional body "arose from the need to regulate standards and provide a network of qualified practitioners with a responsibility to which the public can refer with confidence".

While the associations have tried to systematize the teaching this has not always been entirely successful, partly because the late 1980s and early 1990s also saw the proliferation of associations within certain therapy groups. For example, there are 14 professional associations that represent reflexology. The associations originally emerged from colleges (as in all other therapies that we studied) but in the late 1980s others were independently constructed with more open registers. This expansion has generally served to increase the layers of representation for the reflexologists and potentially confuse the general public.

A further step to identifying commonality across national boundaries has been taken with the establishment of European and international associations and guidelines, a move welcomed by the European Parliament in 1997 as a development towards common standards and regulation of practice. For example, within non-medically qualified homoeopathy, the creation of the European and international councils in the early 1990s marked a commitment to a worldwide core curricula. As the guidelines from the European Council state,

> there should be a comparable standard of education and training in professional *(ie not medically qualified)* homoeopathy throughout Europe and ideally, worldwide. A further goal should be to establish an internationally recognised qualification reflecting this standard (our brackets) (ECCH 1993)

Generally, then, there has been increased agreement on what constitutes minimum standards of education within the majority of therapy groups and many have also moved to produce wider links beyond national boundaries. These developments have not been introduced without criticism, many therapists arguing that the guidelines are too stringent and will cripple innovation. As one homoeopath observed, "I want to get homoeopathy out of this new strait jacket and have something more exciting, so much is being missed out".

Another non-medically qualified homoeopath in Britain, who also acts as a college principal, has refused to conform to the criteria established by the main professional association and has risked losing student applications that are processed via the association.

The tempering of knowledge claims

The early teachings within the therapies often alerted students to the wide ranging potential of their discipline. There was an espousal of the holism of their "art" and a suggestion that other forms of medical care, particularly biomedicine, would become gradually redundant. Within chiropractic, a section of the profession believed that the manipulation of the spine had the potential to cure the whole range of mechanical and organic problems, and in Britain the Druidic homoeopaths stressed the danger of biomedicine, the spirituality of the vital force, and the ability of homoeopathy to deal with all medical problems.

However, throughout the 1980s we witnessed the gradual curtailment of the therapy specific claims, although this may have been accompanied by the expansion of other skills – for example, in the United States osteopaths and naturopaths have acquired skills of general practice (Baer 1984b). In all parts of the world chiropractic has emphasized and developed the musculo-skeletal side of their therapy and jettisoned claims for a wider scope of practice (see Baer 1984b, Willis 1989, Coburn 1991, Cant 1996; also see Ch. 5). As one chiropractor stated,

> by and large it is for musculo-skeletal conditions, areas that the medical profession does not handle very well . . . we used to be alternative to medicine, but now in the UK it's musculo-skeletal and less controversial. Our training has improved and . . . [is] more acceptable to the medical profession (Cant & Sharma 1994).

Moreover, the various groups now perceive their role in the overall health care system to be different. Of course this partly depends on the use of language, but in Britain we have seen the professional associations that represent the various therapies publicly state that their practice should not be regarded as "alternative" but, rather, as "complementary" to biomedicine. This change in emphasis can be seen as a conscious modification to the type of knowledge that is deemed acceptable and the type of public messages that the practitioners are prepared to make. For example, within non-medically qualified homoeopathy, fears that the medically qualified homoeopaths may fight to curtail their practice has led the main professional association to state that homoeopathy should be seen as "complementary" to biomedicine and that the occupation should seek statutory regulation. In a sense, then, there has been a movement away from seeing homoeopathic knowledge as sufficient without recourse to allopathic practices – a tempering of homoeopathic claims and ideals – as the following quotations from one of the Directors illustrate,

> The Directors all say that the Society is ready for complementary medicine, actually working alongside and integrating with orthodox medicine . . . it is the official line.

> We used to have this revolutionary zeal, we were going to replace doctors, but that is bullshit, what will happen, we hope is that GPs will start to be a very sophisticated referral system (Cant & Sharma 1996b: 754).

The latest code of ethics to be released from the Society of Homoeopaths (1997b) outlines areas of competence for the non-medically qualified homoeopath and makes clear that homoeopaths must respect the jurisdiction of their medically qualified colleagues. This includes recognizing that they are not equipped to diagnose and should work towards collaboration:

> The Society recognises that the optimum situation for the patient is one where the homoeopath and the patient's GP establish a sound open and professional relationship . . . whilst current education and training of professional homoeopaths alert the practitioner to the natural progression of disease, it does not equip them to make a full orthodox diagnosis of each and every patient's condition. It is therefore essential that you are aware of the limits of your clinical competence (Society of Homoeopaths 1997b).

This is an issue that has previously stalled talks between the Society and the Faculty of Homoeopaths (the association for medically qualified homoeopaths) and it is hoped that such clear stipulations will encourage co-operation.

It has also been decided by the main professional association that practitioners must no longer advise their patients to reject vaccinations (Cant & Sharma 1996b), previously a very prominent dictum of non-medically qualified homoeopathy, and it is further appreciated that portraying homoeopaths as primary health care practitioners who are capable of treating all illnesses will limit their success. As one of the directors stated,

> Things will not change until GPs know what we can do. A colleague of mine has a very good relationship with a group of GPs. He has agreed on a number of particular problems that he will sort out for patients, things like migraines, but this still depends on the GP wanting to find out what homoeopathy can do (Cant & Sharma 1994).

Thus, the *official* line is that the homoeopaths see themselves in a consultancy role, receiving patients from the biomedical practitioners. Other therapy groups have accepted even more stringent definitions. For example, in Britain the professional associations that represent reflexology have defined the therapy as supplementary to medical practice, expecting not to diagnose or even cure, instead seeing their practice as helpful for relaxation and general healing

(Cant & Sharma 1996a). Clearly this is not a uniform development; for example, in Denmark the reflexologists take on a different conceptualization of their role (Johannessen et al. 1993).

Restrictions have thus occurred in a number of ways. Curtailment can bring contradictions for the therapists, the limitation of the diagnostic claims sitting alongside broad assertions that their practice is holistic. Considering that these holistic principles may be those that attracted patients in the first place, such limitations could reduce the appeal of the therapy and the ability of the practitioner to offer something different.

Alignment to the scientific paradigm

In general we can identify consistent efforts to attach the "complementary knowledge" to the orthodox scientific paradigm, at least in public (such an enterprise is not necessarily followed within the therapies). These efforts have operated at three levels. In the first place, colleges in Britain and elsewhere (Baer 1992) have incorporated medical science into their curriculums and conceive of biology, pathology and physiology as constituent parts of their knowledge system. Such a move has been recommended by the British medical profession (BMA 1993), who have argued that such an education will ensure that practitioners know when to refer patients back to a biomedical practitioner. The professional associations that represent the various colleges also recognize the advantages of medical science. For example, the European Council for Homoeopathy states,

> this component of the course is essential to provide a reference body of knowledge and assessment techniques on which to base safe and competent homoeopathic practice. The programme should offer a common area of concern and communication that facilitates liaison with other health care professionals and enable students to work independently, competently and responsibly within the context of their own national health care system upon graduation (ECCH 1993).

Secondly, the groups have attempted to use orthodox science to try and explain why their therapy works. This has been undertaken in a number of ways, either by drawing on biomedical science or by criticizing medical science and proposing a different scientific paradigm such as quantum physics (see Sharma 1996). For example, chiropractic has applied orthopaedic principles to explain the operation of chiropractic and the homoeopaths have applied a range of scientific principles to explain their approach (e.g. Vithoulkas 1980). Thirdly, complementary medical groups, although this is a hotly contested area, have become more open to the use of scientific procedures, particularly randomized control trials, to establish that their therapy works in practice (Reilly et al. 1986, Meade et al. 1990).

Of course the relationship with orthodox science can be an uncomfortable one. For example, a representative of the chiropractic profession was concerned that using the orthodox paradigm may blinker the profession to new ideas and directions:

> In the 1970s, the pendulum swung from the philosophy of chiropractic to the scientific paradigm. On the one hand this is an inevitable part of the maturation of a profession, getting validation, but it has gone too far, we have lost our openmindedness and our ability to appreciate how things work clinically without scientific evidence, we should not let things go because we do not understand them, or we have lost the next generation of science (Cant & Sharma 1994).

The adoption of the scientific paradigm, in terms of explanation and the use of biomedical diagnostic techniques, also means that many practitioners are using a mix of paradigms. This may be simply pragmatic, as Dale (1996) argues, but has implications for the integrity of certain knowledges and the ways that therapies are understood and developed.

Boundary construction

Originally, as we have seen, "alternative" medical practice was often very open. As one homoeopath stated,

> We had discovered and had been part of a system that was truly wonderful, really and truly wonderful and the fire was there, we wanted to get it to others . . . so that was the motivating force, get it to everybody (Cant & Sharma 1994).

However, there has been a recognition of the need to close off their knowledge. Such closure is made possible by higher entry requirements and longer training programmes – in Britain all the "complete" systems now have courses that span a number of years. Social closure has not been as effective in the other categories, reflexology, massage and aromatherapy, for example, often require short training courses (taught part-time over a few months) and do not demand qualifications on entry.

The establishment of registers of qualified practitioners has also served to demarcate the "authentic" practitioner from those that simply call themselves chiropractor or whatever. By being accepted onto the register, the practitioners have proved that they have passed their examinations and supervised practice and that they have agreed to conform to a strict code of ethics. Any violation of the code of ethics can involve the practitioners being struck off the register and with the introduction of European professional associations the existence of a wider register prevents therapists, in theory, from going and practising elsewhere.

In summary, the last decade has seen a number of changes occur within what might now, in Britain, be termed "complementary" medicine. There has been a general shift to a more stringent form of organization and a more controlled dissemination of knowledge. Furthermore, the content of knowledge has taken on extra dimensions to include those knowledge bases more obviously connected with the biomedical paradigm and its understanding of health, disease and the body. The pluralization (i.e. the expansion) of the available therapies has thus taken place in a context that has required that the therapies conform to some degree to an established paradigm. This is, of course, a generalized picture, one that has identified trends rather than described the specifics within each therapy group. This depiction does mask some of the differences and difficulties that certain therapy groups have encountered (for example, in Britain the non-medically qualified practitioners of homoeopathy have had great problems in coming to any agreement with their medically qualified colleagues) and the fact that a number of practitioners continue to practice in isolation from the professional associations. Nevertheless, both in Britain and elsewhere there is much evidence to suggest that attempts to draw up core curricula, set standards and accredit the knowledge bases of the various therapies is well under way.

Different methods of representation have been chosen, varying from complementary through to supplementary depending on the objectives of the groups and their ability to make a case for their position. For example, the longest reflexology courses in the UK last for nine months, the teaching taking place over weekends at monthly intervals. This length of course is deemed to be sufficient to teach the rudiments of this therapy and does not include extensive discussion of medical science. Consequently, it would be hard to envisage how the professional associations could assert that they work in a complementary way (if such a definition also suggested some degree of equality across the practitioners, rather than simply working alongside the medical profession), and as such they prefer the label "supplementary".

These changes have not been introduced without conflict and many individual therapists are suspicious of the direction that the professional associations have taken. This is particularly the case in our study of non-medically qualified homoeopathy (Cant & Sharma 1996b). There have been concerns around the issues of exclusivity, the loss of the intrinsic qualities of the therapy, the fear of subordination to biomedical authority and practice and the inappropriateness of the scientific paradigm. Those therapists who were involved in the early revival of therapies are often the most concerned and balk at the developments, in particular the idea of restricting the practice of the therapy to a few highly educated individuals, some practitioners suggesting that their practice has become everything that they once deplored. Furthermore, the development of "expertise" is thought by some as contrary to the original principles of a non-hierarchical and participative therapy, with both practitioner and patient involved in the healing process. There are also concerns that the real essence and the individuality of these alternative approaches to medicine have been lost, particularly by accepting a complementary role for their therapeutic practice. Specifically, therapists fear that they may have served to subordinate their knowledge to that of biomedicine. Certainly, while the chiropractors have received statutory regulation (HMSO 1994a), this has not secured them the autonomous position that biomedicine achieved in the nineteenth century, or rights to educational grants, or payment through the National Health Service (see Ch. 5 for more details). On the contrary, their practice is confined to the private sector, their scope of intervention has been defined publicly as musculo-skeletal complaints and they have agreed, in the case of referrals, that biomedical doctors shall retain ultimate responsibility for the patient (Cant & Sharma 1994).[13] Similarly, some homoeopaths feel that statutory regulation will curtail diversity, encourage the re-emergence of a medical monopoly and constitute "sleeping with the enemy" (Kirk 1994:6).

Finally, the alignment to the scientific paradigm has been seen as problematic. For example, some chiropractors feel that the use of orthopaedic science has served to explain away many valuable aspects of their therapy, especially the treatment of organic illness. The homoeopaths still continue to experiment with other bodies of knowledge and in doing so extend their own knowledge (Sharma 1996) but recognize that scientific based knowledge is important for legitimacy and recognition.

The pan-organizational body: the voice of complementary medicine?

If the 1980s saw the shift from individualized practice to schools and therapy specific associations that represented individual therapies, the 1990s saw still further attempts to establish commonality across therapy groups. Within Europe, the potential restrictions to practice that may be ushered in by the European Union have galvanized the development of organizations to represent the interests of the various therapies. These have been national, European and international in structure and have been concerned to scrutinize the credentials of practitioners before putting them on registers, have worked towards common standards of practice and training requirements, i.e. a core curriculum, and the identification of the boundaries that constitute their therapy. Considering the differences that have occurred within single therapy bodies, it is not difficult to imagine the problems that such consolidation has posed.

In Britain, where therapists under the auspices of common law have had the most to lose, the establishment of three separate groups all with the remit to represent the collective interests of therapists was not surprising. The Institute of Complementary Medicine (ICM) was established in 1982 and had as its objectives the dissemination of information about complementary medicine to the general public and the representation of all therapies. In 1989, the Register of Complementary Practitioners was inaugurated which was the first attempt by a national organization to produce a national mailing list and to give assurances that these practitioners were competent to practice. Currently there are 430 organizations affiliated to the ICM (and the ICM has contacts with the awarding bodies of another 500 training courses) and 2,000 (out of an estimated 60,000) practitioners appear on their national list. Despite the wide coverage of the ICM, the British Complementary Medical Association (BCMA) was established in 1990, representing 78 organizations and more than 26,000 therapists, and was the first pan-professional body to produce a code of ethics common to all member organizations. The remit of this group was to cover what they termed "supplementary" therapies such as reflexology and aromatherapy and argues that such approaches should accept a secondary role to that of biomedicine. The BCMA has been particularly concerned to unite the various professional associations that purport to represent a single therapy, for example through the setting up of the Reflexology Organizations Council (ROC) to facilitate talks across reflexology groups. The Council for Complementary and Alternative Medicine (CCAM), represents a smaller number of therapies, those that we might also categorize as "complete" systems, that is, purport to treat the whole range of medical problems (Petrioni 1992).

These associations have had varying success and often duplicate each other's efforts, but the premiss of all three has been to establish levels of agreement across all groups of therapists. The registers are intended to offer the general public assurances about which therapists are safe and trustworthy but, further, are very clear in their portrayal of the therapy groups as complementary or supplementary to biomedicine. The success of the groups has been more about consumer confidence than consolidation of the therapy groups simply because coverage has never been complete and internal arguments about which group has pre-eminence have soured collaborative relations. Moreover, in practice those therapy groups that have undergone the most significant changes in terms of education, state registration, etc. (e.g. osteopathy, chiropractic and homoeopathy) have done so without the help of the umbrella groups.

The reality of being a practitioner

The revival of "alternative" medicine has thus taken on a reasonably distinct format, characterized by layers of organization and increasingly stringent standards. These changes have been undertaken, at least in part, with the intention of enhancing the status and standing of alternative medicine. To fully assess what this new pluralism is like it is instructive to examine the experiences of the grassroots therapists, the extent to which they have personally benefited from the organizational and educational changes and the dilemmas that they have faced.

One way of assessing the experience of the therapists is to focus on the levels of integration with biomedicine. This is an area that we discuss fully in Chapter 6, suggesting that the biomedical profession has retained authority in the treatment and referral of patients. Individual therapists clearly experience problems when collaborating with the biomedical profession, which relate to their proper role, place and position especially if they are employed within the GP premises. The reality is that few practitioners have been able to initiate joint working, and the Society of Homoeopaths has set up a special working party to examine how further integration within the state funded system might be facilitated. The possibility of working in the NHS poses therapists with a dilemma; on the one hand they are attracted to the possibility of security and at the same time are loath to give up the freedom of individual working and the possibility of spending extended periods of time with their patients. Furthermore, in Chapter 5 we discuss the types of support that complementary medicine has received from the state and the implications for working practice to show that while osteopathy and chiropractic have acquired statutory regulation, this has not supplied the therapists with guaranteed work or incomes. In this section we will confine our attention to the social characteristics and financial experiences of the therapists.

It is widely accepted that women outnumber men in the complementary medical market, although the ratios vary by therapy. In our own research (Cant & Sharma 1994) in Britain we found that those therapies, such as chiropractic, that had full-time training and were more scientifically orientated, attracted more men (66 per cent of chiropractors were men in 1994; and in Canada 90 per cent of the chiropractic profession were men – see Mannington et al. (1989)) than in other therapies. Our questionnaires showed further that such practitioners generally had very lucrative businesses, a number of respondents suggesting that they earned over £100,000 per annum. In contrast, reflexology in Britain is dominated by women, less than 10 per cent of the practitioners were men. The study of the membership records of the Society of Homoeopaths, revealed that there were more women in all categories of membership (e.g. student, fully qualified), at least 75 per cent being women, but that the directors of the Society were more likely to be men (in 1995 five out of eight were men). A practice survey questionnaire conducted by this association revealed that the majority of the practitioners who responded earned £5,000 or less per annum. In financial terms, then, for some therapists the salaries are far below those commanded by the medical profession (which can range from £15,230 for a house officer to £43,150 for a consultant), but in the case of chiropractic can surpass the expected medical income (and this is also the case if we compare the salaries to those of physiotherapists). Indeed, for the chiropractors, the possibility of being integrated into the state health service may be financially damaging in view of the salaries they can attract in the private sector. The salaries tended to reflect the working arrangements of the therapist. Chiropractors were more likely to work full time (Mannington et al. 1989) and, in Britain, saw 350 patients per month, usually for 11 minutes each (Huisman 1989, Pedersen et al. 1993).

Explanations for the gender bias are essentially twofold. In the first place it is possible that the therapies are essentially "feminine", incorporating a caring approach to health and healing (this is difficult to substantiate, but see Scott (1998) for a discussion about the feminist nature of homoeopathy). Secondly, it is possible that the alternative medical career is attractive to women because it offers the opportunity for part-time working and consultations fitting in around other responsibilities. It can often be practised from the home of the therapist and need not require extensive capital outlay on equipment. This was certainly an explanation offered by the reflexologists, "It fits in with my life really nicely. I organize the appointments around my children".

On the other hand, this hypothesis is not borne out for chiropractic where in the United Kingdom and America studies have shown that women work the same hours as men (Mannington et al. 1989).

There is very little evidence about practitioners' backgrounds but we can make some tentative statements based on qualitative data collected in 1990 (Sharma 1992) and a very small-scale study of 29 practitioners who worked in one area of England[14] (constituting a response rate of 83 per cent). The questionnaires were sent to reflexologists, homoeopaths and chiropractors and revealed that in the two former professions, practitioners had, without exception, tried other careers before training to be a therapist. By contrast, in chiropractic the age of therapists is generally lower (corroborated by Huisman (1989) who showed the average age to be 39). Communication with the principal of the major college of chiropractic, which now offers a degree, also showed that the college was attracting younger students, straight from school (although most of the recruitment took place in the private education sector as it was felt that these students would have a better chance of securing private funding for their degree programme and may be prepared to invest in the course in the knowledge that later salaries would be substantial).

Motivations for becoming a therapist are hard to generalize. In Sharma's study a number of motivations were identified and included the flexible working practices (deemed to be particularly important by female practitioners); the work fitted in with their personal interests (in particular scepticism towards biomedicine, but also their own illness experience); the desire to help others; and finally the dislike of bureaucratic restraints often found in the workplace, such as hierarchies and organizational formalities. The attraction of occupational individualism may of course be less of a consideration as organizational changes pervade the therapies. Moreover, many therapists felt an uneasy tension between wanting to make a financial living but being able to do so by engaging in a close and caring relationship with their clients. Indeed, there is evidence that many practitioners experience problems in asking for money at the end of the consultation (Sharma 1992) and that patients find the request for money at the end of a confiding session problematic; as one interviewee stated, "it is a completely weird relationship. You tell them everything about yourself . . . he's like a friend . . . and then you pay them".[15]

The role of the therapist can also grant the therapist greater professional powers. Sharma (1992) found evidence of a number of nurses who then retrained in complementary medicine (this is an area that we also discuss in Ch. 4), and found that practising these therapies in the hospital setting did not come under the doctor's scrutiny as other tasks might and thus offered the nurses a degree of autonomy.

Being a practitioner opens doors and causes dilemmas. On the one hand the potential to work in an individualistic and fairly informal manner offers a career structure for many women and in the case of nurses can offer space for autonomous practice. At the same time the salaries are often low and unstable and the contradiction of asking for money can be problematic. Practitioners join their professional associations in varying numbers, probably for insurance purposes rather than for the referral of patients (most patients come through self referral and friends – see Sharma 1992) and many wish the work at a distance from the organizational and ideological restraints imposed by the official representative bodies. Perhaps practitioners are unconcerned about these differences but it is certainly an issue with which the professional associations wrestle, as an editorial in the Society of Homoeopaths journal lamented,

> the present popularity of homoeopathy attracting both patients and those who want to practice it, is a grass roots, bottom up movement. Attempts to regulate it and define it are hierarchical, top-down, so some conflict is inevitable (June 1997, p. 1).

Fission or fusion: implications for the plural market

Generally, although not exclusively, the early stages of the revival of "alternative" medicine can be described as a "cottage" industry – one that lacked organization or central planning, therapists learning their "art" not in training colleges but in their teachers' front rooms or from visits to therapists abroad. The initial re-emergence of complementary medicine was consequently a grassroots, sporadic and disorganized movement. The late 1980s and 1990s have been witness to changes within complementary medicine, especially the inauguration of professional associations, pan organizations and training colleges – what might be seen as the rationalization and bureaucratization of complementary medicine. Such shifts have had implications for the actual shape and form of this plural market.

What can we say about the wider significance of these general changes for complementary medicine? Have the therapy groups acquired greater legitimacy and status and are we seeing a new constellation of interests, a new jostling for position and power in the health care market? Furthermore, if we adopt a postmodernist interpretation that sees a plurality of language games, narratives and social practices, having equal validity, are we now seeing a more even playing field in health care? Or, have biomedical practitioners retained power and authority over other providers? Is there a new big picture for health care? Is there equity or just a new division of labour? When we talk of pluralism are we asking whether there has been a multiplication of health care providers and health care product and the acceptance of many ways of understanding health and illness or are we also interested in their relative power, organization and status?

In the first place, while there has been an expansion in the number of therapies and therapists, pluralization has not simply meant numerical multiplication. At the same time as the field has expanded there have been significant changes in the way that the therapists train, practice and perceive their role. In particular, the coalescence of therapists around common standards of education and the unification into professional bodies has led to a *convergence* in the ways that practitioners train and practice which has acted as a countervailing force to the general pluralization of the market. In other words, the fission and fusion of complementary medicine has occurred simultaneously. Therapies that had publicly stated they had different ways of knowing and treating have, in the first place, taken on board more "orthodox" methods of teaching and practice. In addition, the incorporation of pathology, biology and physiology into the curricula suggests the pervasiveness of biomedical knowledge. Organizationally, there have also been strong attempts to ensure that practitioners share the same educational experience and codes of ethics and consequently the idea of the lone, charismatic and maverick therapist seems less likely. At the level of practice, therapists are seeing their approach at least as "complementary" and are working alongside biomedical practitioners. Of course this may be inevitable if they want the support of the medical profession and state funding, but it also has implications for the ways that the therapists work, not least because of the limited time allowed with patients. Thus, the working practices of complementary practitioners may become more like those of biomedicine. And of course in the current situation, biomedicine retains power and is at the top of any hierarchy that involves joint working, being responsible for the referral or delegation of patients (see Ch. 6). Thus, pluralism involves hierarchical relations in which biomedicine enjoys preeminence. Pluralism, then, is not about equity.

Although we have seen fusion, this has not meant that all the groups have taken the same route and there are distinct differences between therapies especially in the way that they see their role, for example, the reflexologists preferring a supplementary rather than complementary label. And although there has been general pressure to produce educational standards (a pressure not unique to complementary medicine), for some groups coalescence has been easier than for others. Notably, those therapies with shorter training programmes have experienced a more rapid increase in the number of colleges and professional associations. In aromatherapy in Britain for example, there are currently 12 professional associations and 24 training establishments, with a further 67 affiliated training establishments (Baker 1997). This group and others that have experienced a similar expansion (e.g. reflexology) have experienced immense problems in keeping track of all the therapists, never mind ensuring that all members and individual colleges conform to agreed standards. In contrast, in chiropractic, which has a fairly clear constituency with three professional associations and three training schools, the mapping of the profession has been easier (although this did not mean agreement between the three groups was unproblematic or achieved easily: much internal discussion was required before each group would accept working with other therapists who had once stood as their competitors. (See Ch. 5 for more details).

Naturally legitimacy is the goal of all occupations because from it flows all sorts of social, economic and political benefits. To what extent has "complementary" medicine gained legitimacy and how do we measure it? Willis (1989), following Habermas, argues that legitimacy can be sought in two substantive arenas. First, groups can work towards "scientific" legitimacy which is achieved if knowledge claims are commensurate with the scientific paradigm, and attempts are being made at this level. Secondly, "clinical" legitimacy can be achieved and is measured by the extent of use of a complementary therapy by clients and this has been documented in the previous chapter. We suggest that it is also possible to claim clinical legitimacy if the practice has been validated using scientific research methods, whether they be those favoured by biomedical science (e.g. the randomized control trial) or other scientific methodologies. The various therapy groups are now in a position to look at the possibilities of such validation. Furthermore, legitimacy can be secured at an educational level through the acquisition of standards and qualifications. Educational change is not peculiar to complementary medicine; at a time when credentials are becoming increasingly important (Collins 1979), formal schooling and rising levels of educational achievement are a prerequisite to enabling the processes of stratification and the distribution of status. The changes at the educational level do not necessarily ensure higher salaries but they do act as cultural currency that speaks of competency and safety and legitimates knowledge. As we shall see in Chapter 5, some groups have also gained politico-legal legitimacy through state regulation, but such recognition is only available for a minority of groups and does not assure therapists of a strong position in any state funded health care programmes. For all these aspects of legitimacy the groups have needed to be unified and internally regulated and there is evidence of advancement on all these fronts.

Theoretically this poses us with an interesting case study. If we accept the postmodern diversification of knowledge is occurring, it could be argued that we are seeing the revival and growth of multiple ways of knowing about health and illness and how to deal with sickness. However, the ways in which the knowledge of the various·

groups has been publicly transformed tends to suggest that modernist and orthodox standards have been called upon. In other words, we have seen the revival of different ideas and approaches to health care but these ideas have been altered and structured and tied to existing organizational forms and ways of knowing. Such a development has had the effect of marginalizing the complementary medical groups, in that they have lost some of their individuality and have accepted positions of subordination to biomedicine. However, this depiction should not be taken as evidence that the complementary medical groups have sold out or that they have been acquiescent or complacent. On the contrary, as in the case of nurses and midwives before them (Witz 1992), these occupational developments should be recognized as well thought through strategies that have ensured the survival and growth of the therapy groups. The various professional associations have been pro-active, paying attention to contextual demands and pressures and how these need to be combined with their own self interest. The strategies of social closure and credentialism were effective for biomedicine and it is not surprising that complementary groups should choose similar methods to promote their own development. The expansion of complementary medicine has produced a plural medical market, but one where the organizational structures have taken a specific format and where biomedicine has retained, at least for the present time, a position of hierarchical pre-eminence.

Notes

1. Here we suggest that pluralization relates to an increase in the actual number of healing modalities available to the consumer and are not making any comment about their levels of validity and legitimacy.
2. The data comes primarily from a research study in 1992–4 undertaken by both authors, about the professionalization of complementary medicine and funded by the Economic and Social Research Council. We concentrate on non-medically qualified practitioners because their legal position has meant that they have been open to more pressures from regulating bodies and have held a more controversial position in terms of consumer safety and standards.
3. Common law is that derived from custom and judicial precedent rather than statute.

4. Out of 419 students 86 joined the Society of Homoeopaths, the main representative of non-medically qualified homoeopathy in 1991 (the only year for which we could obtain figures) – see Cant & Sharma 1994.

5. Personal communication with Director of the Institute of Complementary Medicine.

6. Wardwell (1994) has demarcated the alternative medical market in the United States into ancillary, limited, marginal and quasi practitioners and has been criticized because these labels come from the relationship that the groups have with biomedicine.

7. Of course for the more established therapies the charismatic beginnings were staged much earlier, e.g. Still and Palmer in the United States and their energetic popularization of osteopathy and chiropractic, respectively.

8. Druids were originally the priests or magicians among the Celts of ancient Gaul and Britain and Ireland. There have always been a small number of people who have claimed to have followed on the Druidic tradition. The leaders of homoeopathy also held chief positions in the Druidic movement.

9. The essential tenets of homoeopathy are contrary to those of biomedicine. Hahnemann's basic idea – *"similia similibus curantur"* or "like cured by like" – involves the prescription of *minute* doses of a substance which, when administered to a healthy person, would produce the very symptoms from which the sick person is currently suffering. The underlying philosophy is that of the *vital force* – that is, Hahnemann believed we are all animated by an abstract form of energy that sustains life but may produce illness if weakened.

10. This was a report, named after the rapporteur appointed to write it, which described the status of non-conventional medicine in Europe and made recommendations concerning education and harmonization.

11. For example, published reports by Consumer Associations such as *Which?* etc.

12. Thus, the majority of students do not join their professional association.

13. This latter principle is also established in the BMA report for all complementary practitioners.

14. This data comes from a pilot questionnaire administered by Sarah Cant in 1993.

15. Taken from interviews with patients of homoeopathy by Sarah Cant in 1996.

CHAPTER 4

Biomedical responses to alternative medicine

The story of biomedical responses to alternative medicine is one of opposition, often virulent, but it is also one of incorporation and accommodation. In this chapter we consider the nature and motivation of these responses and reflect on what they tell us about the changing forms of biomedicine and biomedical hegemony. We shall argue that biomedical responses to alternative medicine demonstrate contradictions in the position of biomedicine – for example, contradictions between holistic aspirations and a reductionist knowledge base, contradictions between an interest in continued professional dominance and the realities of pressures from both "consumers" and the state, and contradictions between the perceptions of various kinds of doctor positioned differently within the health care system.

Historically the medical profession in western countries (as represented by its official national associations) has, in different ways open to it, sought to retain a monopolistic control over the provision of health care. In practice complete control has not been possible; where alternative medicine is not proscribed by law (as in Britain) the medical profession has had limited scope for preventing its re-emergence when consumers are prepared to use and pay for alternative treatments. Where the practice of alternative medicine is forbidden or legally restricted to qualified doctors, the medical profession has more scope to use the law and oppose its relaxation, and has, as we shall see, done so in a number of countries. But given strong popular support for alternative medicines, biomedicine has effectively had to abandon expectations of complete monopoly of the delivery of health care. Medical associations, therefore, have had to concern themselves with retaining and strengthening the role of biomedicine as moral and intellectual *arbiter* of what kinds of alternative medicine are acceptable and legitimate, which conform to good practice, which are efficacious for patients, etc. They have also sought to retain the dominant position of medicine in the therapeutic division of labour so that where forms of alternative medicine can no longer be completely marginalized, they can be brought into the biomedical clinic under the supervision and management of doctors.

We focus mainly on the history of relations between biomedicine and alternative medicine in Britain, paying special attention to the development in the late 1980s and early 1990s of a more accommodating response and we try to account for this shift. (We deal mainly with expressed attitudes in this chapter; the issue of practical co-operation with alternative practitioners is dealt with in Ch. 6.) As we shall indicate, in other western countries the story has not been identical; the therapies that evoked greatest medical ire or anxiety have not everywhere or always been the same, and the stakes for the medical profession have depended much on the local form of the alliance between state and biomedicine.

Neither biomedicine nor alternative medicine is a simple unitary entity. Each is a complex of different groups and interests. It was always the case that some doctors practised medicine regarded as unorthodox by their peers, indeed some forms of alternative medicine were developed by people institutionally rooted in the biomedical profession of their day. (Radionics, for instance, was originated by Dr Albert Abrams, an American professor of pathology.) Neither biomedicine nor alternative medicine are unchanging categories and, considered as bodies of knowledge, they are not necessarily mutually exclusive or invariably structurally opposed.

Nonetheless, biomedicine constituted itself as a moderately unified professional grouping much earlier than did most forms of alternative medicine. From the mid nineteenth century in Britain (and from around the same time in most other western countries) it enjoyed an increasingly close relationship with the state. The 1858 Medical Act granted doctors state registration for the first time and in doing so laid the foundations for an alliance between biomedicine and the state which was to grow and strengthen, with the medical profession gaining the status of a privileged "insider" group (see Ch. 5 for a more detailed account of this relationship). This Act also contributed to the very definition of the boundaries of biomedicine itself, for it established the General Medical Council which had oversight of the content and scope of medical curricula and training.

In contrast, the forms of healing regarded as unorthodox by biomedicine have emerged at different times and have their own peculiar histories. The very notion of "alternative" medicine as a generic category towards which the medical profession might have an overall response is a recent one.

In eighteenth-century Britain the invective of medical men against "quackery" disguised a state in which, from the point of view of the public at any rate, the "quacks" and the "regulars" might not have been easy to distinguish. At this time any kind of medical practice depended much on the ability to attract and keep patients through reputation and perceptions of therapeutic success on their part (Jewson 1974). In this consumer led market, the patronage of the wealthy and influential was crucial. Regular medicine (if by that we mean the treatments offered by those practitioners licensed by the Royal Colleges) does not appear to have enjoyed the kind of therapeutic success that would have made it the automatic choice of all or even most patients who could pay for treatment. All medicine was commercial to an extent and the genteel public appears to have been fairly well informed about what was available and about the ideas and knowledge on which it was based (Porter 1985). "Regular" medicine could only with difficulty appeal to some kind of self evident moral or practical superiority over other available forms of healing.

The term "quackery" implies professional dissimulation, deliberate deceit of the public on the part of charlatans without any proper training or real knowledge. In the circumstances, doctors could really only either attack individuals on the basis of the falsity of their peculiar claims and remedies, or inveigh against quacks in general on the grounds of their charlatanry. Neither the knowledge of the doctors themselves nor that of their competitors constituted well ordered and consistent systems of professional knowledge as yet, so medical criticism was directed at individual practice rather than theoretical underpinnings. Although the scientific understanding of the working of the human body advanced rapidly during the eighteenth century, this knowledge had yet to revolutionize practical everyday therapeutics. Nor were the therapeutics of the "quacks" based on recognized bodies of theorizing. From this point of view, Porter is right when he suggests that these healing practices conducted by individual entrepreneurs in pre-nineteenth century Britain were not the direct ancestors of the main forms of alternative medicine we see today. The "quacks" might have claimed to be better and to have more effective remedies or even to be morally superior to the "regulars", but Porter doubts whether seventeenth and eighteenth century "quackery" constituted a "mutiny" against orthodox medicine based on an alternative knowledge base and epistemology (Porter 1989:129).

Particular schools of unorthodox healing emerged at various times in the nineteenth and twentieth century, each with its own distinct knowledge base and an identifiable (if not always very coherently organized) collectivity of practitioners. Biomedical attacks on the unorthodox then shifted from invective against "quackery" to critiques of the "unscientific", and "science" increasingly served to define the boundaries of a profession that sought to impose its own definition of valid healing practice. In the following section we offer an illustrative outline of how biomedicine has responded to three well known therapies.

Biomedical strategies of marginalization. Homoeopathy, acupuncture and osteopathy

Homoeopathy

Homoeopathic medicine became popular in England in the second quarter of the nineteenth century, a time when regular medicine relied much on the administration of "heroic" remedies, the use of venesection, violent purgings, strong sedatives such as opium, and other forms of treatment – drastic and usually highly unpleasant in their immediate effects. Homoeopathy, in contrast, took a minimalist approach, administering highly dilute dosages thought to stimulate the patient's "vital force", whose weakening is the basic cause of all illness. However homoeopathy was not a separately organized profession at that time. Homoeopaths were doctors who operated within the existing provincial medical associations. In the second half of the nineteenth century, as the alliance between medicine and the state was beginning to be forged, there began what Nicholls has called the "ostracism" of homoeopathy (Nicholls 1988:133ff. See Ch. 3). Within the medical profession, bitter attacks were mounted on those practitioners who also practised homoeopathy. These discreditation strategies included the critique of statistics that suggested the positive benefits of homoeopathy. There were also attempts in the 1850s to have homoeopathic physicians charged through the law courts with the death of patients whom they had not succeeded in curing (Nicholls 1988:147). It was argued that the principles on which homoeopathy was based were absurd and that homoeopaths were either under some kind of delusion or were fraudulently practising medicine which they knew to be ineffective. Yet at the same time there was a creeping incorporation of some homoeopathic remedies into the regulars' repertoire and the adoption of more allopathic techniques by the homoeopaths, who also began to de-emphasize the more controversial teaching of Hahnemann (especially the theory of the vital force). Nicholls calls this the "bastardisation of homoeopathy" (Nicholls 1988:165ff). Homoeopathy as practised by the doctors trained in the Faculty of Homoeopathy in London became a tolerated if insignificant and marginalized group within the broader medical profession, and when the National Health Service was established in 1948, homoeopathy was grudgingly accorded a foothold within it.

During the 1970s we see the medically qualified homoeopaths starting to wage their own campaign against non-medically qualified homoeopaths who emerged in Britain at this time. The Faculty's newsletter at this time sees the discussion shift from how to make homoeopathy more popular with other doctors to how they should deal with the lay "threat". Again, the basis of the attack was discreditation – the non-medically qualified homoeopaths were berated for their dangerous lack of medical training and their emphasis upon the metaphysical. Medical homoeopaths took a renewed interest in the scientific vindication of their therapeutics – not so much through proof of the basic theory of homoeopathy as through clinical trials of particular remedies. In this way they could distance themselves from the "non-scientific" homoeopaths.

Associations of sympathizers and users of homoeopathy were a feature of homoeopathy both in Britain and elsewhere (Wolff 1992), a means by which doctor homoeopaths rallied support in the face of threats from the medical profession and spread knowledge about homoeopathy. They now used such channels for warning their own partisans and the public at large of the dangers of treatment at the hands of the medically ignorant, though this did not make a great deal of difference since the non-medically qualified used the same strategy and formed a partisan support group of their own, the "Friends of Homoeopathy". In summary, homoeopathy in Britain had been marginalized by the medical profession to the extent that the main dialogue was now between the doctor homoeopaths and the non-medically qualified homoeopaths (with some signs latterly of *rapprochement*).

Acupuncture

Acupuncture originated in China and is established as an orthodox mode of treatment there, a generic therapy which can be applied to the whole range of medical conditions. It spread sporadically and slowly beyond China throughout the eighteenth century (Saks 1995:110ff) and was practised by medically and non-medically quali- fied practitioners in the United Kingdom in the early part of the nineteenth century. On the whole, acupuncture as "naturalized" in Britain was divested of its classical theoretical underpinnings in Chinese diagnostics and understandings of the human person. From the mid-nineteenth to mid-twentieth century there was what Saks calls a "climate of rejection", medical journals showing little interest in the therapy and denouncing non-medically qualified acupunc- turists. This seems to have been a matter of indifference as much as professional hostility. There was no institutional equivalent of the Faculty of Homoeopaths within the medical camp and doctors wishing to learn acupuncture had to teach themselves or attend private colleges (Saks 1995:125). But for the same reason there was no titanic struggle *within* medicine between the proponents of the therapy and its opponents.

Recently the practice of acupuncture as a limited technique within medicine has become more acceptable within the biomedical profession. It has been regarded as particularly useful in the treatment of pain, and medical acupuncturists have made various attempts to interpret this effect in terms of orthodox medical theories about the nervous system (Fulder 1996:133). Medical acupuncture has been compartmentalized to the extent that it is used for a restricted range of conditions. But this very compartmentalization has served to distance doctor acupuncturists from the growing body of non-medically qualified acupuncturists who practise acupuncture as a more generic therapy and who regard themselves as more faithful to the original Chinese therapeutic tradition.

The response of organized medicine to acupuncture in Britain seems to have been much colder than in many other European countries such as France and Russia, where it is now taught in medical schools and can almost be thought of as part of the mainstream biomedical canon. As Saks argues, the reception of acupuncture in the West has varied greatly between different societies. However incorporation into the medical repertoire in countries like France or the USA does not mean that practice of acupuncture by non-medically qualified practitioners is any more tolerated by doctors there than it is in Britain.

Osteopathy

As a result of interest in rehabilitation and orthopaedics after the First World War, osteopathy (founded in America by Andrew Still, 1824–1917) began to gain some popularity in Britain. Medical opposition to this competing modality intensified in 1920s. A bid for state registration was made by osteopaths in 1931. The response from the medical profession stressed both the lack of empirical evidence for the existence of the "osteopathic lesions" posited by Still and the unsatisfactory nature of osteopathic training and qualifications. To the latter claim the osteopathic profession was indeed vulnerable (Larkin 1992:122). The developing alliance between the medical profession and the Ministry of Health in the 1930s led to the blocking of several further attempts at state registration. In 1935, 800 medical and biological scientists signed a statement submitted to a Select Committee of House of Lords, stressing the lack of scientific evidence for osteopathic theory of lesions and the British Medical

Association made a submission stressing the incompatibility between osteopathic and modern medical concepts of the nature of pathogens.

In the USA, where it originated, osteopathy had a rather different history and by the Second World War had actually achieved a degree of convergence with biomedicine to the extent that in 1963 the US Civil Service Commission declared that the MD (medical) and DO (osteopathic) degrees were to be regarded as equivalent. This was the culmination of a process by which the American Medical Association effectively sought to "tame" osteopathy by assimilating it into biomedicine (Gevitz 1988b).

In Britain, the story was to be acceptance with subordination rather than acceptance with amalgamation. After the Second World War there was a greater tolerance of osteopathy by British doctors, some of whom practised it themselves. They may have been influenced by the growing awareness that in Britain chronic back pain was a major problem accounting for much distress, not to mention loss of days at work, to which biomedicine had only limited answers. By this time British osteopathy itself had become a more restricted modality, with less grandiose claims, increasingly specializing in a limited range of musculo-skeletal problems (though some osteopaths may have privately regretted these limitations. See Sharma 1995:181). While the 1986 British Medical Association (BMA) report on alternative therapy (see below) gave only very grudging recognition to osteopathy, the various surveys of doctors' attitudes, to which we shall refer later, showed that many doctors held a much more positive view. Recognizing this, there was a radical shift in official attitudes. The Osteopaths Act, providing state registration, was passed by Parliament in 1993 with the approval of the medical profession, who were widely consulted (Kings Fund 1991:35). Once osteopathy had relinquished its claims as a generic form of medicine, and once it had achieved a form of professional organization acceptable to the medical profession, it was no longer seen as a threat but as a modality that could usefully supplement medical care in the difficult area of musculo-skeletal problems.

In this brief and highly selective review we have seen that, prior to the 1970s, the most aggressive medical attacks on non-orthodox forms of treatment have taken place when a particular therapy has seemed to be gaining competitive ground in a particular area or areas, or to pose some quite specific kind of threat to the plausibility of the medical profession's practical dominance. Medical responses have taken the forms of discreditation, exclusion, mobilizing support to block legislation, professional marginalization of doctors practising alternative therapies, resort to law. However they have also included selective incorporation or acceptance of some techniques and procedures, where these could be fitted into and subordinated to the structure of the biomedical clinic.

The specific modes of opposition and the outcomes of these struggles, as we have seen, have been diverse. One could argue that while homoeopathy was marginalized, acupuncture was selectively incorporated and osteopathy was tamed. In the cases of homoeopathy and acupuncture the situation was complicated by the presence within the medical camp of doctors practising the therapies themselves, albeit in a different fashion from non-medically qualified practitioners (some doctors practice osteopathy but they are less visible as a group within the medical profession). Much has depended on the claims made by the therapies. Those with less generic aims (such as reflexology) have attracted little attention from the medical profession as measured by, for example, articles in the scientific medical press. However there have been considerable national differences in medical responses to individual therapies. Acupuncture was more readily incorporated in France, and chiropractic – eventually accepted in much the same way as osteopathy in Britain – engaged in a long and bitter struggle with the medical profession in America (see below).

Biomedicine from the mid nineteenth century to the 1970s was far from being an inflexible and unchanging entity. It was capable of responding to non-biomedical therapies that challenged its attempts to monopolize therapeutic provision and authority. It did this by taking on aspects of those therapies doctors regarded as useful and which could be incorporated into medical practice (as in the case of acupuncture) and opposing that which it could not assimilate. What it did not tolerate was organized and articulate professional groups (whether within or outside its own ranks) who promoted tenets or practices at variance with those that were the basis of its own dominance.

However alternative medicines were not perceived as a generic threat until the revived popularity of older therapies, which began to be evident in the 1970s, and the arrival of many newer therapies on the scene. There now emerged a more generic response to alternative medicine on the part of the medical profession. While there continued to be distinct responses to specific therapies there developed a sense that the therapies constituted some kind of collective phenomenon, a more general challenge to medical dominance and authority.

Alternative medicine as a generic issue

In Britain, the legal position regarding non-biomedical therapies has always been liberal. The 1858 Medical Act did not prevent therapists without medical qualifications from practising within the law, provided that they did not claim the title of medical doctor. However the attitude of the medical profession itself was more restrictive and until 1974 the General Medical Council (GMC) ruled that doctors who collaborated with unqualified practitioners of any kind might be struck off its register (Fulder 1996:88). There has been no modification of the principle that a doctor who delegates treatment to a non-medically qualified practitioner of any kind must be assured that the practitioner is competent to undertake the treatment, and must retain overall therapeutic responsibility for the patient. Strictly speaking, therefore, while alternative practitioners may "refer" patients to doctors, doctors cannot "refer" patients to an alternative practitioner (or not in the same sense), only "delegate" treatment as they might to a nurse or a physiotherapist, retaining diagnostic control and ultimate clinical responsibility for the patient.

From the late 1970s, however, alternative medicine emerged from a period of relative quiescence and became a source of collective anxiety for the biomedical profession, and not just in Britain. First, there was the arrival of new therapies such as reflexology and aromatherapy, and the increase (among both old and new therapies) of practitioners who had not undergone any kind of medical training and whose 'qualifications were unfamiliar to the medical profession. Secondly, there was the increased "consumer" interest in alternative medicines documented earlier (see Ch. 2). General practitioners, in particular, became aware that their own patient lists must include some of these users. Studies of doctors' perceptions of alternative medicine began to report consciousness of a "demand" for these therapies on the part of patients – either a general demand or specific requests for referral directed to GPS themselves (65 per cent of doctors responding to a survey in Canada reported that they perceived a "demand" for alternative medicine; Verhoef 1996. See also Himmel et al. 1993 for data from Germany). Practical anxieties were expressed in the national and international biomedical press. If patients under medical treatment used forms of alternative medicine which were actually dangerous, how could doctors stop them and how could they take any responsibility for what happened to such patients? How could a doctor ever be satisfied that the therapist had genuine qualifications and competence? (Murray & Shepherd 1988:514). If patients feared to admit to their doctors that they were using non-biomedical treatments (as was clearly often the case) the potential problems were even greater (Elder 1997).

These anxieties were expressed in the context of a more general insecurity about extremely well informed patients, in possession of more information then ever before about medical matters through the media. Patients were expecting to participate more in decisions about treatments, and were more liable to challenge medical decisions and diagnoses (Blair 1985) or even enter into litigation. As it became evident that many AIDS patients (especially in the USA) were experimenting with non-biomedical treatments of one kind or another, there was anxiety that patients might not be able to distinguish between alternative clinics which offered something useful, if no more than a sense of empowerment, and those which promoted "worthless or even harmful treatment" at great expense (Greiner 1995:178–9).

One biomedical response was to stress the potential or actual dangers of unproven alternative treatments. Risk might arise directly from treatments which could cause physical harm to the patient. Herbal treatments, such as the internal use of comfrey (Whitelegg 1996) and some Asian forms of medication used by hakims from the Indian subcontinent, came in for particular attention in Britain (Kew et al. 1993), with much stress being placed upon the toxic potential of some of the substances used. While there is no reason to suppose that such dangers are not very real, especially where patients are dosing themselves unsupervised, the evidence of people actually coming to harm in this way was of its very nature anecdotal, i.e. just the kind of evidence that doctors were ruling as inadequate when adduced in favour of alternative treatments.

A second kind of supposed danger could arise more indirectly when a patient with a life threatening condition delayed consultation with a medical doctor by wasting time on ineffective treatment from an alternative therapist. Again, there was little evidence that this was a widespread problem, indeed research on usage showed that it was unusual for patients to make the alternative therapists their first port of call; most people consulted only after they had already tried conventional medicine and found it, from whatever point of view, unsatisfactory for their problem.

Another biomedical response was an ever greater emphasis on the need for scientificity. Specific therapies had already come under fire for their lack of scientific validation. This was now discussed as a generic issue. Command of scientific expertise and professional morality are explicitly linked in a 1983 *British Medical Journal* editorial which urged doctors to assume the role of discriminating guides for patients attracted by the apparent benefits of alternative healing regimes:

> At the heart of the matter is the reality that the public sees doctors as scientifically trained clinicians; and that means they have a professional obligation to help guide them through the claims and counterclaims of practitioners on the medical fringe. Uncritical enthusiasm has no place in such an evaluation; the crucial tests are the objective ones (Smith 1983:307).

Similarly, Skrabanek, in a critique of acupuncture claimed the approach had no scientific validity and that acupuncture ignored the "demarcation between science and quackery, between reason and faith, between an honest search for truth and unscrupulous exploitation of human suffering" (Skrabanek 1984). (Note the conflation of scientificity and professional altruism in these quotations.)

More than this, it was now feared that there was a general turning away from science itself – it was the patients' lack of confidence in science that was the issue as much as the therapies' lack of scientificity. Thus a 1980 *British Medical Journal* editorial entitled "The Flight from Science" explicitly linked alternative medicine with consumerism, medical litigation and what it saw as a scaremongering critique of modern medical treatments and technology:

> ... in medicine the results of consumerism have been damaging and will continue to cause harm until risks and benefits are put back into balance ... Our objections to the claims of the chiropractors, and to the critics of the drug industry, of intensive care or coronary thrombosis, of obstetrics and indeed, of ortho-dox medicine are not – as they often suggest – a reflex reaction by a defensive autocratic profession. No: what is wrong is the refusal by the critics and the fringe practitioners to accept the standards of proof that medical scientists have developed in the past hundred years; not for nothing has the concept of the randomised double blind controlled trial been described as one of Britain's most important contributions to medicine since the war. (*British Medical Journal* 1980: 1)

The lack of scientificity of alternative medicine itself is here seen as linked to a general public defection to irrationality and superstition. At this time there were signs of official anxieties about what was broadly termed "the public understanding of science". Govern-ments often justify their actions in terms of the "scientificity" of the information on which they claim to act. In 1990 British Junior Health Minister Stephen Dorrell declared that he needed good "scientific" evidence of the efficacy of complementary therapies before the government could recognize them (Thomas 1990a). If this form of legitimation is to work, the moral standing of science in the eyes of the general populace has to be a matter of concern.

The "alternative" critique of modern biomedicine could be dis-missed on the intellectual grounds of unscientificity but politically it could not be ignored by national medical associations. In 1983 Prince Charles, then President of the British Medical Association (and like a number of other people in high places, known to take an interest in alternative therapies), urged doctors to take a critical look at their apparent lack of holism. In the same year the BMA set up a working party to look into the claims of alternative medicine and to evaluate its potential usefulness.

The working party consisted entirely of people from the bio-medical establishment, with a heavy presence of pharmacologists. The document they produced in 1986 is in some ways extraordinary.

The first 34 of its 161 pages consisted of an account of the progressive development of modern biomedicine as a scientific discipline, with a lengthy disquisition on the statistical techniques used in clinical trials. Some of the main forms of alternative medicine were then discussed, with an assessment of any scientific evidence for their efficacy. The general conclusion reached was that there was insufficient evidence for doctors to feel confident about the prospect of recommending alternative medicine to patients or of working more closely with therapists. The appeal of alternative medicine, the report argued, was understandable in view of the fact that its practitioners often had more time to provide the compassionate empathy which many patients needed and found lacking in hard pressed NHS staff. But patients must be protected from treatments that are not scientifically validated and may even be harmful:

> While we have a duty of fairness to the practitioners of alternative therapies, our long term duty to our patients is not to support what may be passing fashions, but to ensure for them the benefits of medicine in the future. These include future applications of scientific knowledge: but also, and just as important, orthodox medicine carries the safeguards which arise from entrusting the preservation of health and the care of disease to a registered, recognised and accountable profession, with a long standing tradition of scientific and personal integrity, including strict standards of confidentiality (BMA 1986:76).

Here again is the appeal to the moral as well as the scientific credentials of biomedicine as safeguards for the "vulnerable" public.

The 1986 BMA report was taken by the therapists and their supporters as evidence of just how intractable were the barriers that alternative medicine was up against.

Medical support for alternative medicine

Doctors' attitudes: survey research

The very negative tone of the 1986 BMA report must have been perplexing to some doctors. The period that produced the "Flight from Science" editorial and saw increased stress on scientificity as a boundary marker for the biomedical profession, not to mention the first BMA report, also saw the publication of a number of surveys showing a high degree of interest in alternative medicine among doctors. David Taylor Reilly's study of young doctors showed that 21 per cent practised some form of alternative medicine and 80 per cent would like to train in one or more form of alternative medicine; a third claimed to have referred patients for treatment by hypnosis, manipulation, homoeopathy or acupuncture (Reilly 1983). In Wharton & Lewith's study of GPs in Avon, 38 per cent of respondents claimed to have some training in some form of alternative medicine, 15 per cent wished to arrange training in one or more technique, and 76 per cent had actually referred patients to some form of alternative medicine (chiefly spinal manipulation, hypnosis and acupuncture) during the previous year (Wharton & Lewith 1986).

It is likely that respondents in such surveys tend to be those doctors who are already favourable to alternative treatments, others being less inclined to spend time on filling out questionnaires on the subject. However, it is still worth noting that only 16 per cent of Anderson & Anderson's respondents defined alternative medicine as "unscientific", and only 3 per cent of the respondents in Wharton & Lewith's study thought that alternative practitioners ought to be banned (though 93 per cent felt that they should be regulated). These studies do not reflect the hostility or dismissiveness shown in the "Flight from Science" editorial, nor do the respondents seem to have been greatly perturbed personally by the lack of scientific evidence for the therapies they favoured.

Having said this, we must bear in mind that most of the questions in these studies invited respondents to give their reactions to specific therapies rather than to "alternative medicine" in general. As we might expect, the respondents displayed different degrees of interest in different therapies, manipulation acupuncture, hypnosis and homoeopathy evoking the greatest interest. Disciplines such as herbalism and reflexology evoked much less interest and/or were less positively evaluated. We should also point out that respondents to these questionnaires often made the distinction between medically qualified practitioners of alternative medicines and those without medical qualifications. Finally, while many respondents in these studies claimed to make use of some form of alternative medicine in their practice, there is no evidence that such practitioners had any very thorough training in alternative therapies, or that their knowledge was more than superficial, an issue which surfaced in the second BMA report (see below).

The juxtaposition of research findings of this kind, and the strictures of the first BMA report reveal an apparent disjunction between the views of many ordinary GPs and those of the official spokespersons of their profession. The 1986 BMA report calls for randomized control trials, yet Nicholls & Luton's local study reveals a community of GPs as sensitive to demands posed by changing attitudes to alternative medicine among the public at large as to the demands of science: "It would appear that the lay world is able to exert some effect on the content and judgement of professional discourse" (Nicholls & Luton 1986:13). This may be more than just a form of medical populism however since Nicholls & Luton also point out that both "medical and patient interest in alternative medicine relates to its ability to provide effective curative or palliative treatment with respect to historically specific profiles of disease" especially "intractable morbid conditions unresponsive to medical intervention" (Nicholls & Luton 1986:14). That is, alternative medicine is perceived as treating exactly the kind of conditions which GPs routinely encounter, rather than the kinds of condition likely to be familiar to the specialists and pharmacologists who constituted the BMA working party.

Studies comparing doctors working in different contexts might reveal whether GPs are indeed a special group in terms of their attitudes to complementary medicine. We have only encountered one such study, a recent survey by Perkin et al. (1994) which compared GPs, hospital doctors and pre-clinical medical students in respect of their attitudes to and knowledge of five complementary therapies. This certainly showed a lower level of interest in and use of the therapies on the part of hospital doctors, but the differences were not large (e.g. 20 per cent of the GPs were treating patients by using some form of alternative medicine as compared with 12 per cent of the hospital doctors). A Canadian study suggests that factors other than location within the health system may be relevant; female GPs were more favourably inclined to alternative medicines than male GPs, and place of training was also influential (Goldszmidt et al. 1995).

Data from other western countries suggest a very widespread groundswell in favour of *rapprochement* with at least some types of alternative medicine. Ernst's meta-analysis of studies of doctors' attitudes to alternative medicine in a range of countries (north European, New Zealand, Israel) suggests that the level of approval for some alternative medicines is high, at any rate among general practitioners. The manipulative therapies are the most popular among doctors, with acupuncture and homoeopathy ranking next. The level of interest was also fairly consistent between different countries – in general the majority of respondents in these surveys expressed positive attitudes to at least one form of alternative medicine. However, as Ernst points out, these results need to be interpreted cautiously since it is difficult to say how far such surveys obtain a representative medical view, and there are differences in methodology between the surveys which make comparisons difficult (Ernst 1995).

Ernst's view is that doctors' perception of the usefulness of alternative medicine as evidenced in these surveys "differs substantially from proven effectiveness as supported by randomized controlled trials" (Ernst 1995:2406). While medical scientists and the official voices of the biomedical profession call for more scientific testing of alternative therapies, a large body of general practitioners in many western countries are clearly not waiting for medical researchers to endorse alternative medicines before they refer their patients to it or practice it themselves, a contradiction of which the BMA report makes no mention.

Another way to look at the issues is less in terms of the differences between actual groups of doctors, and more in terms of the viewpoints of different kinds of medical knowledge. Pickstone has distinguished "biographical" medicine as the medical knowledge derived from the observation of the effects of disease on particular bodies, encountered in the context of the life courses of given individuals. Biographical medicine may draw on generalizeable principles, but it observes these principles as they manifest themselves at work in individual patients. From this point of view "anecdotal" evidence about the course of a particular patient's disease or cure (important in the generation of many kinds of knowledge in complementary therapies) may be highly significant. This kind of knowledge is contrasted by Pickstone with the analytic knowledge of hospital based medicine, the experimental knowledge of the university laboratory and what he calls "techno-science", characteristically generated by industrial companies (Pickstone 1993).

The biomedical critique of alternative medicine mounted by the BMA in the 1980s celebrates these latter approaches with its stress on the randomized double blind clinical trial, in which it is not the subjective responses of patients that are recorded and monitored but "variables". The 1986 BMA report makes no mention of the biographical medical knowledge which has great practical importance in most areas of therapeutics (nowhere more so than in general practice). The distance of holistic alternative therapeutic knowledge from the experimental knowledge of the university and the large scale trials of the pharmaceutical laboratory was thus amplified, and the commonalties of holistic alternative practice and the general practice of biomedicine were made invisible. The attack on alternative therapies was made by glossing over a contradiction within the biomedical camp, a tension between different kinds of biomedical knowledge, which was becoming difficult to ignore.

Holism in biomedicine

Holism as a therapeutic ideal can be understood in a variety of ways, the common factors being regard to the patient's subjectivity and treating sickness as more than a set of physical symptoms (Sharma 1994:86ff). The biomedical version is probably as much influenced by psychoanalysis, via the work of Michael Balint (Balint 1957) as by specific theories about the unity of mind/body/spirit. Paradoxically, an explicit commitment to holism in biomedicine among doctors begins to manifest itself at the very time when the official medical critique of alternative therapies intensifies. Medical critics of alternative medicine are fond of claiming that biomedicine, in its ideal form at least, does attend to the whole person; alternative practitioners have no monopoly on the notion of holism (e.g. BMA 1986:75). But if the holistic ideal was a bone of contention for some, for others it created a bridge. The British Holistic Medical Association (BHMA) was founded in 1983 by Patrick Pietroni and has been first and foremost a biomedical association, with GPs as the largest category of members. The BHMA was from the outset well disposed towards the practice of complementary therapies within

medicine. It has a category of membership for complementary practitioners and its newsletter carries a good deal of information about
seminars and training opportunities in complementary therapies.

At the very time when the BMA was lauding the historical development of objective scientific knowledge in medicine, the biomedical holists were stressing the mind/body link, the importance of the
patient's own subjective experience, the need for compassionate
physicians to heal themselves. Such values encouraged a more
open outlook. A typical attitude was that expressed by Dr Richard
Morrison, writing in the BHMA newsletter about the experience of
running a course in physical examination for homoeopaths:

> Although the medical profession has tended historically to be
> rather possessive about its body of knowledge, this now seemed
> an anachronism, and the sharing of information between disci-
> plines a more positive and constructive attitude – provided we
> all recognised the limitations of that information and used it
> responsibly (Morrison 1990).

That this recognition of limitation was not always easy in practice
becomes evident when we look at accounts of collaborative projects
(see Ch. 6). However, some GPs were evidently becoming acutely
aware of the contradictions between (on the one hand) the ideal of
the caring practitioner who knows the patient and the context of his
or her sickness, and (on the other) the joint effect of the reductionist
approach to the body inherent in modern technological and scientific biomedicine, and the pressures of an underfunded public
service with less and less time available for the individual patient.

Other professional groups

The negative response of the BMA can also be contrasted with the
more welcoming attitude of the nursing profession. A survey of
readers of the *Nursing Times* showed that more than half of
respondents had used complementary therapies of some kind in
their work, mainly massage, aromatherapy, reflexology and shiatsu.
These were used mainly for stress reduction, pain relief, insomnia,
pregnancy and labour, and palliative care (Trevelyan 1996:42). The
Royal College of Nursing established an official interest group for
complementary medicine (the Complementary Therapy Forum) in

1993. This group now has over 2,000 members who practice some form of therapy, although the majority use the therapies as an adjunct to their work (i.e. spend less than 80 per cent of their time on them). Most use the "tactile therapies" which involve shorter periods of training and which do not make wide generic claims (D. Rankin-Box, pers. comm., 1997).

The appeal of these forms of alternative therapy for nurses is not difficult to see. Nurses tend to be more patient centred in their practice and see themselves as encouraging patients to take responsibility for their care. Nurses commonly lay claim to holism and are liable to distinguish their work on the wards from that of hospital consultants on such grounds (Williams 1989). Models of the nursing process that stress the acceptance of the interdependence of the physical, spiritual and environmental aspects of patients' lives, and a desire to place greater emphasis upon the process rather than the outcome of care, have become more prominent, both in Britain and America (Watson 1995). McMahon has shown that the key features of the nurse–patient relationship – those of intimacy, reciprocity and partnership – are also crucial to complementary medicine (McMahon 1991).

One can also interpret this interest in terms of the changing professional project of nurses. Just as doctors assimilated acupuncture into their body of knowledge to limit competition it is possible to see nurses' adoption of complementary skills as providing them with another area of expertise, one where they can claim special knowledge and discretion, thereby potentially enhancing their professional status. As Rankin Box points out, clinical nursing practitioners are actively seeking to utilize specific therapies and to lay claim to their use as specialisms within their professional remit (Rankin-Box 1993).

Doctors do not seem to have regarded this apparent expansion of nurses' competence as a threat to their own professional position, probably because it does not seriously disturb the original biomedical division of labour. Nurses practising at their own initiative are generally using therapies like aromatherapy or reflexology, regarded by doctors as innocuous provided that they do not make diagnostic claims. They are also unlikely to conflict with treatments prescribed by the consultant. In general practice, the doctor can delegate limited complementary treatments (e.g. some forms of acupuncture) to a suitably trained practice nurse without any abrogation of therapeutic responsibility or control. Indeed such delegation may save the doctor valuable time, especially if the nurse can use the time with the patient as an opportunity to offer lifestyle advice and emotional support (Hubble & Middleton 1995:173).

Complementary therapies are also enjoying great popularity with midwives and physiotherapists, no doubt for very similar reasons to that of nurses. However, in all these professions it is recognized that complementary medicine offers opportunities that call for proper training and standardization. There are potential issues of accountability, responsibility and interprofessional communication and boundaries (Marshall 1995).

Into the 1990s: contradictions in biomedicine exposed

The British Medical Association (again)

Possibly the BMA subsequently comprehended the extent of the contradiction between the grassroots assessment of alternative medicine by ordinary GPs and that of its 1986 working party. Possibly they realized that changes in the NHS made the incorporation of some alternative therapies into the NHS inevitable. In any event, in 1990 a second BMA working party on alternative medicine was set up, with a rather different composition. This time it included a GP and was advised by Dr D. Taylor Reilly, a doctor qualified in homoeopathy who had carried out clinical trials of homoeopathic remedies. This working party had the remit "to consider the practice and use of complementary medicine since 1985 throughout the UK and the European Communities and its implications after 1992". The introduction to the report, far from decrying consumer interest in complementary medicine, frames the project squarely in the context of providing suitable medical guidance to the consumer:

> It is not, therefore, the place of the medical profession to proscribe the legitimate activities of consumers in health care. However doctors have a duty to the individual and to the community to safeguard the public health and to this end, it is important that patients are protected against unskilled or unscrupulous practitioners of health care. It was therefore

considered helpful for the BMA to consider as a *public health* issue, the principles of good practice in non-conventional therapies which would safeguard the individual against possible harm to health and maximize the potential benefits of particular methods (BMA 1993:2).

The language is no longer that of scientific proof of efficacy, but that of accreditation, competence to practice and consumer protection. The substitution of the term "complementary medicine" for "alternative therapies" was in itself considered significant, suggesting as it did the possibility of co-operation and the recognition of what had been seen before merely as "therapies" as forms of "medicine". In its recommendations the working party did, to be sure, reiterate the call for good research on proof of efficacy but paid much more attention to the issue of proof of practitioner competence. It called for regulatory bodies to be set up for each therapy with registration procedures, well defined areas of competence, enforced ethical codes and proper complaints procedures, agreed standards of training, etc. Significantly, it recognized the need for protocols for co-operation between doctor and complementary practitioner; provided that standards of competence were laid down and maintained, the GMC might now consider permitting doctors to refer patients to therapists (in the sense of passing on to them the responsibility for diagnosis and decisions about treatment) as opposed to the delegation of specific treatments, which was already permitted. This was a very significant shift from former positions, as also was the recognition that doctors practising complementary medicine without proper training might be as dangerous to the patient as non-medically qualified therapists.

We could interpret this as a radical U-turn on the part of the representatives of the medical profession. Alternatively, we could see it as something far less radical – the shift from a celebration of the *cognitive* authority of medicine as a form of scientific knowledge to a celebration of its *moral* authority to protect the consumer by pronouncing on standards of competence. If we take the second view, then medicine has not admitted a concession of authority – only shifted the grounds on which it claims this authority.

In any case, whatever the public position of the BMA, it would be highly misleading to suggest that biomedical opposition to alternative medicines had been entirely eroded. One might even argue that there was something of a backlash in some quarters. Medical scientists now challenged alternative medicines to demonstrate the efficacy of their interventions through the kind of empirical testing that medical science recognizes, the Randomized Controlled Trial; no reputable professional could honestly purvey "unproven" remedies, and indeed biomedicine itself was under greater and greater pressure to practice "evidence based medicine". In the next two sections we examine two *causes célèbres* which illustrate the nature of this backlash.

The Campaign Against Health Fraud and the role of the pharmaceuticals

In 1989 the Campaign Against Health Fraud (CAHF) was launched in Britain, a partnership between medical researchers and investigative journalists claiming to protect the vulnerable patient against the claims of those who peddled unproven treatments. The CAHF, given the facetious sobriquet "quackbusters" by some, claimed to be there to "bust" any kind of health fraud (whether alternative or biomedical) and that the principle of *caveat emptor* could not be applied in the field of health care. The advocates of alternative medicine saw the campaign as an arrogant manifestation of medical reductionism, conducted by doctors interested only in drug treatments, unconcerned with the iatrogenic damage done by many of those selfsame treatments (Martin 1989). Furthermore, they resented what they saw as an attempt to arrogate to orthodox medicine the responsibility to put the alternative therapies' house in order (Editorial, Journal of Alternative and Complementary Medicine, June 1989).

In fact the main targets of the Campaign Against Health Fraud, which later changed its name to the more innocuous sounding "Healthwatch", appear to have been nutritional treatments, whether practised by biomedical or alternative healers, which used vitamin supplements and the like for conditions such as cancer, allergies, and ME, and other regimes that might conflict with important drug treatments currently being researched.

This raises the general question of the role of pharmaceutical companies. The precise nature of whatever links existed between

CAHF and commercial interests is unclear. Caroline Richmond, a journalist who was one of the leading activists in the CAHF, was apparently permitted to use the address of the Wellcome Foundation for mailing campaigning letters, and CIBA allowed the use of their premises for the newly formed group to hold its first Steering Committee meeting. Some leading medical members of CAHF were researchers who had known links with pharmaceutical companies through research grants (especially with Wellcome) or with other commercial interests, notably food processing companies (Walker 1993:335). It is not at all clear whether the campaign itself was directly funded by any of these organizations. Members were evidently sensitive to the accusation that this might be the case, and the issue of what kinds of donation the CAHF might accept was debated at its AGM in 1990. The minutes recorded that no money had been received from any pharmaceutical company, but the meeting voted that donations might be accepted from such sources provided that they were on a strictly "hands off" basis (Walker 1993:339). CAHF did eventually achieve charitable status.

In 1993, journalist Martin Walker published a book entitled *Dirty Medicine* which claimed to reveal the links between the pharmaceutical companies (and other commercial interests) and the attacks that the CAHF mounted upon alternative medicine and "natural" health care. Walker gives detailed accounts of the involvement of CAHF in such issues as attacks on the opponents of the controversial AZT drug for the treatment of AIDS patients, or in hostile campaigns against treatments for allergic conditions based on "provocation neutralization" rather than drug therapy (promoted by doctors such as Dr Jean Munro of the Breakspear Hospital). The evidence adduced by Walker for a link between drug companies and the CAHF is mainly circumstantial; he does not provide data to prove conclusively that direct transfers of funds took place, or that there was explicit briefing of CAHF members by Wellcome or any of the other bodies implicated. However there is plenty of evidence in the book for what he calls their "tacit support" (Walker 1993:646). The matter of the means by which the same bodies actively supported the promotion of drugs like AZT in the face of growing scepticism on the part of the patient community and those who represented them is a different case, and Walker has much to say on what he sees as the dubious research ethics of some of the trials which medical scientists used to test drug based interventions, and on some of the "dirty" tactics used by the CAHF and others in the medical establishment to discredit individuals who opposed the use of drugs from one point of view or another.

In April 1994, Duncan Campbell, the journalist who was a prime mover in many of the activities that Walker claimed to have exposed, wrote to the *Journal of Alternative and Complementary Medicine*, which had recently published a favourable review of Walker's book. Campbell suggested that Walker himself had been paid large sums of money from unspecified sources to research and write the book and accused Walker of threatening and unprofessional behaviour (Campbell 1994:4). The editor published an apology to Campbell and withdrew support for the book. The necessity of this was evidently disputed by a number of readers of the journal, so in the June issue the editor published a more detailed justification for his action which indicated that he himself could attest to certain inaccuracies in Walker's accounts of events in which he himself had been involved: "The fact is that while some of *Dirty Medicine* may be correct, some of it is not, and I will not defend what cannot be defended, from whatever side of the holistic divide it emerges" (Chaitow 1994:4).

It would take a major effort of investigation to discover exactly how much of the book can be regarded as reliable. Given the importance of the issue, it is extremely unfortunate that the first major attempt to research the links between opposition to alternatives to drug therapies and commercial interests was apparently flawed. The links which Walker claims to have uncovered are all too plausible.

However, supposing that we reserve judgement on the absolute accuracy of all that he writes, what do we learn from Walker's book that is relevant to our purpose? His material suggests that the main targets of CAHF/Healthwatch have been practitioners who have promoted nutritional treatments for conditions such as cancer, AIDS, allergies, ME, etc., or who have espoused other therapies that conflict with drug treatments currently available or being researched. Many, if not most of these have been qualified doctors with an orthodox medical training who, doubtful of increased reliance on drug based interventions, have developed alternative regimes in their (mainly private) clinics and hospitals. CAHF appear to have evinced much less interest in individuals practising systems such as reflexology, oste-opathy or acupuncture in a general way, i.e. those who do not use medication and who do not make claims in respect of certain condi-tions or diseases.

It is quite possible that the pharmaceutical companies do not see alternative medicine in general (as opposed to specific treat-ments) as a major threat to their interests. Some may even see the re-emergence of alternative therapies as a new opportunity for profit. In Britain, Boots launched a new range of homoeopathic remedies and its retail stores have begun to sell a variety of herbal and other "natural" remedies. British expenditure on non-conventional medicinal products amounted to £66 million in 1994–5 (Gordon 1995). Some Swiss companies have taken an interest in the work of herbalists, offering the possibilities for the development of new drugs from recently discovered constituents (Jain 1995).

The re-emergence of alternative medicine has actually created novel commercial opportunities. Some US health insurance com-panies own holistic clinics in spite of opposition from the American Medical Association (Lagnado 1996). This trend has reactivated existing commercial interests in alternative medicine itself, which was never without its own material products and medications. Many alternative treatments (e.g. Vega testing) involve the use of complex equipment which must be manufactured and marketed by some company or another. In the same year as Walker's book was pub-lished, a controversy erupted in the pages of the *Journal of Alterna-tive and Complementary Medicine* (*JACM*) about a decision on the part of the British School of Osteopathy to produce a booklet in co-operation with Crooke's Healthcare Ltd. Crooke's are the manufac-turers of the analgesic Nurofen, and the booklet was to promote Nurofen as an adjunct to osteopathic treatment. The British School of Osteopathy accepted funds from Crooke's to finance student bursaries for osteopathic training (*JACM* February 1997:7). Com-panies who manufacture natural health products have been active in campaigning on behalf of natural medicine; the Research Council for Complementary Medicine acknowledged sponsorship for its newsletter from Lambert's Dietary products and from Larkhall Laboratories (RCCM 1989:2) and in its annual reports openly pub-lishes lists of companies and trusts from which it has received donations.

Biomedicine clearly has its commercial allies, but the general relationship between capitalist interest and therapeutic activity is a complex one. The problem with Walker's investigation is probably not so much a matter of the accuracy of detail as an underestimation of the flexibility and responsiveness of modern capitalism to new markets and opportunities. Wellcome and CIBA may well back opposition to specific drugs in which a great deal of research effort and marketing has already been invested, but in the end it may be less of a problem for multinational corporations to transfer funds and research energy to new forms of medical product than it is for medical researchers entrenched in a particular outlook and professional context to abandon their commitment to reductionist understandings of the body and to the kinds of scientific testing which these understandings predicate.

One of the most important products of medical scientists' participation in debates about alternative medicines has been the reiteration of calls for the subjection of "unproven" interventions to the "gold standard" test, the RCT. These calls have become more insistent, notwithstanding the more relaxed attitude of the BMA and notwithstanding the ethical and scientific flaws revealed by Walker and others in the conduct of some of these very trials. The scandal of the research into the Bristol Cancer Help Centre in 1990 showed what a large methodological beam some medical scientists needed to remove from their own eyes before they criticized the unscientific motes in the eyes of other people.

The Bristol Cancer Help Centre furore

In September 1990, an article was published in the *Lancet* which convinced many proponents of alternative medicine that opposition from medical quarters was still deeply entrenched (Bagenal et al. 1990). This article was an interim report on data from a study carried out by the Imperial Institute for Cancer Research at the invitation of the Bristol Cancer Help Centre (BCHC), a clinic offering natural and holistic treatments and dietary regimes for cancer sufferers. The study compared women who had had treatment for breast cancer at the Centre with breast cancer patients who had followed orthodox treatments. It appeared to show that the women using the Bristol Cancer Help Centre had poorer chances of survival than those who used orthodox treatments, seemingly confirming those medical critics who saw alternative treatments as (at most) making people "feel good" in the absence of any proven clinical change in their condition.

The appearance of this report, much publicized by the media, created shock waves among those who had been sympathetic to the use of alternative medicines to treat or support cancer patients, and demoralized many of the patients themselves. The Bristol Cancer Help Centre's waiting list numbers dropped dramatically and its insurance cover was threatened (Thomas & Bishop 1990:10). The substance and implications of the report were widely debated in the medical press. This debate revealed what would not be evident to someone who had read only the sensational press reports and not the article itself, namely that the methodology of the study was seriously flawed. More detailed discussions of the faults in the research can be found in Thomas & Bishop (1990), Stacey (1990/91) and Stacey (1991), but the main issue was the design of the study which did not compare like with like. The patients at the Bristol Cancer Help Centre were (by definition) a self selected group so there was no possibility from the outset that the study referred to a genuinely randomized trial of methods of treatment. Nor was there a full exploration of other factors that might make such patients different from the subjects who had not experienced BCHC treatments. For example, BCHC patients were likely to have had cancer longer and to be at a more advanced stage (most had only come to Bristol after receiving extensive orthodox treatment first). Nor was there any investigation of whether the Bristol patients were actually compliant with the various regimes recommended to them at the Centre. Some critics also pointed out that the study not only threw no light on the causes for the differences in outcome between Bristol patients and the "control" group, but that it could not even be said to be looking at the relevant differences. The ICR study looked mainly at survival, whereas some critics suggested that, given the therapeutic goals of the Bristol Cancer Help Centre, enhancement of quality of life was more important. The research team itself was somewhat divided as to the significance of what they had published. In the end Dr Clair Chilvers, the Professor of Epidemiology at Nottingham University who had led the research, expressed regret that the study had been taken to indicate that the Bristol regime itself was responsible for difference in survival rates, and admitted that the differences found were as likely to be the result of the more advanced state of the disease in the Bristol patients.

A common perception in the alternative medicine world was that it was too early to expect a fair and objective trial to be conducted by a team of orthodox scientists, and that medical scientists had no right to lecture alternative therapists on the need for rigorous testing of treatments when many medical procedures have never been properly tested on biomedicine's own terms (Stacey 1988). However the issue of scientificity and proof of efficacy remains an active one and is likely to remain so with the general insistence on "evidence based" medicine, even if institutional obstacles in the way of co-operation between alternative practitioners and well disposed doctors are being eroded (an issue which we deal with in more detail in Ch. 6).

If the collective voice of the British biomedical profession seems to have taken a less strident tone towards alternative medicine of late this has not meant that biomedical opposition has disappeared. It has meant, rather, that biomedical opponents have caught a glimpse of the limits of their institutional power to reverse the growth of alternative medicine when it is popular with patients, has established an holistic market, has some influential advocates from within the medical profession itself (such as Dr Pietroni), when there is neither legislation that can be brought into operation nor (as we shall see in the next chapter) any great governmental will to interfere with this growth. In this situation, biomedical critics of alternative medicine direct their energies much less to explicit opposition to the attempts of well organized professional groups of healers to obtain legitimacy and recognition. The critique now focuses on the "unproven" nature of many alternative interventions and the need to devise and conduct the right sort of reliable scientific trial. Many of those whose professional interests and activities place them in the "alternative" camp concur with the need for scientific trials of alternative medicines and procedures. The Research Council for Complementary Medicine, for instance (founded in 1983), has had as its object the promotion of scientific research on alternative medicine and has done a great deal to bring together alternative medicine and medical science. Established medical scientists have found work for themselves in this field: Professor Michael Ginsburg, former Dean of Basic Medical Sciences at King's College, was the Consultant in Research Development for the RCCM for some time, and a German medical scientist, Edzard Ernst, was appointed Professor of Complementary Medicine at the University of Exeter. There is a small but steady stream of publications on scientific trials of alternative medicines in the biomedical press.

It is an interesting reflection of the ways in which things have changed – and at the same time not really changed at all – that an article by Professor Michael Baum, a founder member of CAHF, appeared in *Complementary Therapies in Medicine* (journal of the Research Council for Complementary Medicine) entitled "What is holism? The view of a well known critic of alternative medicine". In this article Baum applauds holism as a worthy scientific and therapeutic ideal; holism reflects the hierarchy of levels at which the human organism operates and can be studied. This hierarchy enables Baum to distinguish between interventions that address the molecular level and those which address the broad relation between consciousness and the organization of the material systems of the body.

> Complementary medicine is practised at the highest level, that is at the hierarchy that governs the human organism. Providing it avoids the temptation of using its notions and potions at lower levels in the hierarchy, e.g. cells, it is saved from the hazards of reductionism. Providing the complementary physician concentrates on making the patient feel better and spiritually at ease, then its position is secure into the new millennium. I would also urge proponents of complementary medicine to appreciate that the holistic system is an open system which lends itself to the experimental method. There is much research required to investigate the psychosomatic aspects of disease and the spiritual dimensions to healing. Complementary therapists, therefore, should resist complacency and join forces with clinical scientists to explore the domain between the mind and the neuro-endocrine levels of the human organism (Baum 1998:44).

We have quoted at length from this piece because an article that starts out by deploring the limits of scientific reductionism in medical research practice turns out in fact to be a celebration of this very approach. Alternative practitioners should concentrate on areas where the placebo effect can be activated, but interventions that address the biochemistry of the body are the province of medical science. Yet the study of this very placebo effect requires that alternative practitioners school themselves in experimental science. What appears to be a rather disarming admission of the limits of medical science is no less than a warning to alternative medicine to keep its hands off areas that are the preserve of the medical scientists or at least to recognize the primacy of the scientist's expertise in the investigation of therapeutic effects.

Medical responses: a comparative view

So far we have concentrated on Britain, but is this a typical case? Not only does Britain have very liberal laws on alternative medicine, but the majority of its doctors are directly employed by the state and therefore, it could be argued, enjoy a high degree of professional security and protection from the effects of competition.

There is sufficient consistency between the ways in which biomedical doctors are trained and practice in different countries for the notion of biomedicine as a transnational entity to remain valid and useful. Yet the institutional position of biomedicine is not the same everywhere. The differences that are most relevant to biomedicine's reaction to the resurgence of alternative medicine include, as we have seen in the case of Britain:

1) the nature of the relationship between biomedicine and the state and the kind of privileges which this position has accorded to doctors in terms of income, status and opportunities.
2) the context of the biomedical clinic consequent upon this state/biomedicine relationship, in particular whether biomedical doctors practice primarily in a market or quasi market situation or whether they practice in a public sector that protects them to some degree from the direct expression of patient demand.
3) the historical legal position of biomedicine, especially the extent to which national legislation restricts or prohibits the practice of alternative therapies by persons other than biomedical doctors.

These are only the broad dimensions of difference. As we saw from the British case, the undoubtedly dominant position of doctors *vis-à-vis* other kinds of health care professional does not mean that the context in which biomedical doctors practice is stable or that they can take the basis of their power for granted. In Britain the introduction of an internal market in the NHS, and the subjection of clinicians to more managerial and budgetary control has not dislodged them from a position of enormous privilege compared with other health care professionals, but it has led to a situation where many doctors feel (negatively) more exposed to new currents of patient expectation while some feel (positively) more able to argue for the buying in of certain kinds of alternative medical expertise into NHS contexts.

A major difference between the situation of biomedicine in Britain and that in many of its European neighbours has been the historical legal situation. In countries in which legislation has restricted the practice of healing of any kind to biomedical doctors, the medical profession has been able to use the law in a way that was not open to the medical profession in Britain.

In France, for example, the medical monopoly over the legitimate provision of health care has a much longer history than in most other western countries and the relationship between the state and the medical profession has been closer and more direct. French law prohibits the practice of medicine of any kind by persons not trained as doctors. Homoeopathy and acupuncture are however widely practised by doctors themselves, and the law has not prevented a large number of lay practitioners of various therapies from flourishing in recent years (Bouchayer 1991).

Bouchayer reports a loosening up of official medical attitudes to doctors practising well established forms of alternative medicine (Bouchayer 1991:50). But at the same time, she says, there is increased vigilance against doctors practising what are regarded as more doubtful therapies, and more doctors are appearing before professional disciplinary boards. And though the practice of alternative medicine by lay persons continues to be widespread, doctors who do not regard alternative medicines as benign have been very active in taking individuals to court for the illegal practice of medicine. A case in 1993 concerned a lay homoeopath in Fayence, Provence, accused by a local doctor. The homoeopath mounted a defence on the plea that he did not practice nor did he claim to practice "medicine" as such. His patients, he argued, came to see him of their own free will and received written advice about which remedies they might use. He did not provide them with a prescription for medicines which could be reimbursed by the state. (Gordon 1993:17). If doctors are to continue to attempt the control of alternative practitioners through the exercise of the law, then the issue of what constitutes "medical practice" in French law may turn out to be a crucial one.

However, while the law is otherwise unequivocal as its stands, the effect of the market situation of doctors balances the effect of their legal strength. Various pressures (notably perceived over-supply of qualified doctors) make the practice of a therapy like homoeopathy very attractive to the doctor who is seeking a specialism in order to obtain patients in a very competitive climate (Laplantine & Rabeyron 1987:67). As Traverso found in a study of doctors who practised acupuncture or homoeopathy, such practitioners situate themselves firmly and clearly within the medical profession, albeit distancing themselves from tendencies (overuse of drugs treatments, lack of attention to the patient's perspective, etc.) which they feel have denied the humanistic promise of modern medicine. (Interestingly, in view of what was noted earlier with regard to differentiation of medical attitudes to complementary medicine, Traverso's interviewees saw hospital consultants as among their most serious adversaries within the medical camp (Traverso 1993:192).)

In strong contrast to France, biomedicine in the USA achieved its privileged position in relation to the state and to other forms of healing much later and in a different fashion. As in many European countries, the general social legitimation of biomedicine emerged through legislation in the various states concerning who could practice which forms of healing, but also through the decisions of insurance agencies, through which much health care is funded, as to which non-biomedical treatments (if any) they were prepared to reimburse.

A situation something like that described by Porter for eighteenth-century Britain persisted for much longer in the USA. A wide range of healing modes flourished in nineteenth-century America, especially in the frontier areas where the absence of a good supply of regular doctors meant that many forms of unorthodox practice flourished in an unregulated market. The American Medical Association (AMA) campaigned vigorously against what it regarded as irregular medical practice, but it was not until after the promulgation of the Flexner report on medical education in 1910 that the marginalization of these forms was assured. The Flexner report advocated a stress on scientific training and privileged the forms of knowledge and education used by biomedicine. As a result of these reforms many colleges which had offered courses in homoeopathy and other popular forms of medicine could not obtain the private funding on which American training colleges largely depended. Those that survived, like many of those offering training in osteopathy and chiropractic, managed to do so because their curricula approximated more and more closely to the biomedical curriculum (Baer 1992). In addition, the American Medical Association decided to grant licensure only to those medical schools approved by its Council of Medical Education.

The relationship between the state and the organized medical profession was never as direct as that which obtained in France. However the AMA had a strong influence on legislation regarding health practitioner qualifications and licensing arrangements in general (Salmon et al. 1980). Paradoxically, in spite of ideological conditions much more favourable to the philosophy of the "market" than in either Britain or France, and a consumer ideology of "free choice" in medicine, many American states passed restrictive laws that actually forbade the practice of specific forms of alternative medicine (Sale 1995).

Yet one could argue that the situation in the United States has demonstrated the propensity of the medical market to enter in "by the back door" where ideological conditions favour enterprise and are antithetical to public provision of health care. As Goldstein suggests, the American medical culture has always allowed a good deal of latitude to the individual physician as regards style of practice and clinical decision-making, permitting a degree of responsiveness to the demands and preferences of patients. Generalizing about the United States is risky since different states have different legislative provision and there are many other local variations, but physician referrals to alternative practitioners would seem to be common, generally on the basis of patient demand (Borkan et al.

1994). There is, as in Britain and the other countries we have considered, widespread practice by medical doctors of certain forms of alternative medicine and a recent report listed 29 medical schools offering courses to medical students about alternative medicines, mainly as a result of student demand (Pavek 1995). As in Britain, a holistic tendency in a certain section of the medical profession is very conspicuous, especially among primary care physicians, and there has been an American Holistic Medical Association since the late 1970s.

We do not need to conclude from this, however, that the legitimation of alternative therapies has been or will be a smoother process in the USA on account of a more market oriented ideology. We find articles in the medical press showing the same attitude of cautious and rather sceptical detachment expressed in much British medical writing, presenting alternative medicines as something physicians need to know about because their patients are likely to use it or demand it, rather than because of its intrinsic merits (Murray & Rubel 1992). And we also find the prototype of the British "quackbusters", the National Council against Health Fraud, apparently waging outright war against non-orthodox methods of treatment (Baran et al. 1993). This group has had no compunction in using restrictive state laws where these exist to bring cases against individual practitioners. And where state laws define the "practice of medicine" in such a way as to exclude such modalities as homoeopathy, doctors have not been slow to bring cases against "deviant" colleagues, as in the case of Dr Guess, a family doctor found guilty of unprofessional conduct by the North Carolina Board of Medical Examiners for prescribing homoeopathic remedies.

On the whole the American Medical Association (unlike the BMA) seems not to have attempted to develop a prescriptive overall view of alternative medicines on behalf of its members and the public at large. Where the American medical profession did mount a very prolonged and focused crusade, however, was in the case of chiropractic. This therapy is thought of in Britain as primarily a manipulative modality which, like osteopathy, is particularly suitable for musculo-skeletal problems. However chiropractors in the USA were early on divided into two camps – the "straights", who regarded themselves as holding to the pure tenets of Palmer, the founder of chiropractic, and the "mixers" who were to become the majority. The mixers adopted a more eclectic approach, adding a number of other modalities to their chiropractic skills. In America and Canada chiropractic developed into a highly popular form of healing. American chiropractors, especially the mixers came to treat a wide range of medical problems and for a time seemed to be offering a service nearer to that of a general practitioner (Baer 1982). Indeed, from the point of view of the straights, their practice and training seemed to have taken on a great deal of biomedical knowledge and the distinctiveness of chiropractic was thereby diminished.

The services of the mixers were, however, very popular and the number of chiropractors grew in spite of medical opposition This popularity was reflected in their statutory position. There are laws for the licensing of chiropractors in all of the states and reimbursement of chiropractic fees is possible under the Medicare insurance programme (Cobb 1977). Chiropractors achieved this position in the face of determined opposition from the AMA, and Coburn & Biggs suggest that the chiropractors succeeded in America and in some other countries because they did not attempt to obtain a secure position through persuading doctors to plead on their behalf. They effectively bypassed the patronage of the official medical professional organizations, building on their general popularity to put direct pressure on legislators (Coburn & Biggs 1986:1036).

The medical profession in America remained bitterly opposed to their claims, on the grounds that the theory of chiropractic had no scientific basis, nor was there scientific evidence for its therapeutic success (Coulehan 1985). This continued even at the time when doctors in the USA were demonstrating a more relaxed attitude to therapies such as osteopathy. In 1976, five chiropractors brought a case against the AMA and ten other medical organizations under American anti-trust law, claiming a conspiracy to prevent doctors from associating professionally with chiropractors. All the other organizations accused settled out of court, but the AMA was eventually found guilty of criminal conspiracy and obliged to revise its policies. As a result of this ruling chiropractors now have a status which is much higher than such specialisms enjoy even in Britain, where they are among the alternative therapies most favoured by doctors. They can for instance obtain hospital posts and use hospital diagnostic facilities. On the other hand, unlike osteopaths (who have a status in the USA much nearer to that of an MD) chiropractors seem to be evolving into a

> limited medical profession, limited to treating the neuro-musculoskeletel system using principally spinal manipulation together with a restricted range of adjunctive therapies, primarily physiotherapy modalities (Wardwell 1994:1066).

The case of chiropractic is of particular interest and we have discussed it at some length since it demonstrates what we have already argued in the case of Britain, namely that the stiffest medical opposition is aroused by those therapies that compete most closely with biomedicine in terms of whom they serve and what they do. Organized medicine is less likely to devote a great deal of energy in opposing what (from their point of view) are the more bizarre and outlandish therapies if their practitioners do not compete with it for legitimacy, funds or patients.

The difference between the USA and Britain lies less in the nature of the "backlash" effect evidenced in CAHF, and such activities, as in the nature of the contradictions that have been exposed by the popularity of alternative medicine. In Britain, and in western countries in general, alternative medicine exposed, and indeed benefited from, the contradiction between biomedicine's aspiration to provide a personal and even holistic professional service to the patient and the increasing reductionism of its scientific base. In the United States, a further contradiction was exposed between the liberal ideology of the free market (which was popularly held to apply to medicine in America in a way that, post 1948, had been rejected in Britain) and the actual monopolistic tendencies inherent in much professional and commercial practice in advanced capitalist economies. In the case of biomedicine these tendencies were actually supported by legislation restrictive of healing practice by non-biomedical practitioners in many states.

However the British case is somewhat unusual in terms of the speed with which the professional body representing biomedical doctors retreated from an explicitly oppositional view in the face of alternative medicine's surge in popularity, and the way in which direct opposition and lobbying was left to individuals or to pressure groups like CAHF. In Sweden, for instance, the legal situation has been even more liberal with regard to non-biomedical healing practice than in Britain. Attempts to clarify the position of non-orthodox healers took place much earlier than in most other North European countries with the passing of an Act in 1915 which actually removed the monopoly of the medical profession by leaving the door open for traditional healers, the only form of health care available to people in isolated rural areas. Though more restrictive legislation was passed in 1960, government attitudes have been generally more positive to alternative medicine than was the case in Britain, where as we shall see in the next chapter, governments took a somewhat "hands off" approach to the issue until very recently. But the Swedish Medical Association took a much more antipathetic view of the manipulative therapies than did the medical profession in Britain (Eklöf 1996:192). Unlike the BMA, it opposed legislation for the state registration of chiropractors (passed in 1994) on the grounds that the benefits of manipulation were not scientifically demonstrated, that adequate training for chiropractors was not yet available in Sweden, and that in any case professions already registered (doctors and physiotherapists) could already provide adequate treatment. After the event there was much disgruntled reference in the medical press to "political pressure". Eklöf has traced a highly oppositional stance on the part of the medical profession, as evidenced both in terms of official statements and in terms of contributions to medical journals, discourse which proposes a need to keep biomedicine "clean" from the taint of unorthodox practices. As in other countries where the official organ of the medical profession explicitly opposed the attempts of alternative therapists to gain greater legitimacy, this official stance was not reflected in the practice and attitudes of many ordinary doctors. For example, a recent questionnaire survey of doctors showed that 66 per cent of doctors thought that chiropractic was an effective treatment, and more had agreed that legislation to register chiropractors was desirable. As in many other North European countries, doctors in Sweden have begun to co-operate with practitioners of chiropractic, homoeopathy and naturopathy, and some practice homoeopathy and anthroposophical medicine themselves (Eklöf 1996, Eriksson 1993:60).

Discussion

There is not so much a single biomedical response to alternative medicine as a range of responses; different kinds of doctor have different kinds of stake in the quasi monopolistic status of biomedicine and doctors do not regard all alternative therapies in the same light. What our discussion has shown, however, is that the resurgence of alternative therapies has exposed and exacerbated certain contradictions within biomedical practice. One such contradiction is that between biomedicine's own "scientific" claims and aspirations to a caring personal service. Another is the institutional contradiction between its claims to moral and professional authority and the fact that it is more and more exposed to market or quasi market situations in which the "purchaser" has some measure of control over what is offered, or how it is offered, limited though this measure of control may be.

We have also seen that the resurgence of alternative medicine raised questions about boundaries. The aggressive attitudes we have described do not relate solely to fears about the erosion of whatever degree of monopolistic privilege biomedicine enjoys locally, but to anxiety about where the line is to be drawn between biomedicine and other forms of healing. Some national medical associations have tried to police the use of unconventional therapies on the part of their members (see Dew 1997 for an interesting case from New Zealand) with varying success. Medical researchers have represented experimental science as their shibboleth but, as we have seen, many GPs in Britain and other countries are eager to practice some alternative treatments, in spite of their efficacy never having been proven through RCTs or other kinds of rigorous testing. GP biomedical practice has probably always been pretty eclectic – GPs in Britain, the USA and elsewhere are not so far removed from the eclecticism of the mixer chiropractors which the AMA so relentlessly attempted to eliminate. The notion of science as boundary marker is harder to maintain in these conditions.

But alternative medicine is also a highly complex grouping. The story we have told suggests that we have to ask whether or not there is a constant entity called "alternative medicine", to which the medical profession can be deemed to "respond". In some periods, and in some kinds of discourse, doctors have dealt with "quackery" or "alternative medicine" as generic types. At other times and in other situations doctors have been careful to differentiate between the types of non-orthodox medicine, castigating some as unscientific while even co-operating with the practitioners of others.

In most of the countries we have examined, a period of generic resistance to alternative medicines following their rise in the 1960s and 1970s was very quickly succeeded by a period during which, whatever official professional attitudes were maintained, local hierarchies of acceptance were effectively worked out; in many European countries one or more of the manipulative therapies has come to occupy a high and relatively less controversial status in relationship to medicine (osteopathy in Britain, chiropractic in Britain, Sweden and Switzerland). Homoeopathy as practised by medical doctors has a similar status in France. In most western countries there is not a simple binary division of health care into "orthodox" and "alternative". Standing between the orthodox medical profession and the "fringe" of practices that are well beyond the medical pale there is a privileged group of relatively well regarded therapies having some degree of statutory recognition or security. So the category "alternative medicine" is always the rather ambiguous and shifting product of a configuration of popular and medical attitudes, legal and official definitions at a given time and place.

Most sociological analyses have dealt with medical attitudes to alternative medicines in terms of professional self-interest (Easthope 1993, Saks 1995). This concept is fine as far as it goes. We could hardly begin to understand, say, the story of American doctors' opposition to chiropractic without reference to it. But if it is our only instrument of analysis it proves to be a rather blunt one, since there is virtually nothing that doctors might do in relation to alternative medicine that could not (*post hoc*) be attributed to professional self-interest. If organized medicine rejects alternative medicine this can be construed as an attempt to defend medical monopolies, but if individual doctors start to practice it then this is also professional self-interest – doctors act in this way so as to add to their repertoires and not lose patients. Appealing to professional self-interest does have the advantage of helping us (if we need such help) to see through the rhetoric of altruism used by doctors in relation to alternative medicine. We have seen how medical construction of the vulnerable patient enables doctors to cast themselves in the role of protectors of the public from the claims of unregulated (or even unscrupulous) therapists. It is also, as Saks points out, an improvement on the cruder versions of arguments to the effect that "holism is opposed by doctors because it is against the interests of capitalism" (Saks 1995:140ff).

The notion of self-interest has more analytical value if we take into account the fact that it is not always material interest which is at stake. Biomedicine in western countries still has great prestige and is well paid, notwithstanding theories about deprofessionalization. There is a growing rather than a shrinking demand for medical services. However the stakes today are less the number and patronage of patients than the moral position which doctors have achieved as a result of their various kinds of partnership with the state, as arbiters of what is sickness and what is not, of who is deserving of treatment and who is not, as protectors of the public against fraud and quackery. It may be that it is the possible loss of moral authority in the face of the claims of alternative medicines to be more caring and more patient centred that is the greatest threat to professional self-interest. This danger has to be seen in context of the diverse other "challenges" which have been made to the authority and therapeutic expertise of biomedicine in recent decades – increased medical litigation, the growing role of self-help groups, public doubts about the safety of drugs, the critique mounted by feminists, etc. (Gabe et al. 1994).

But the interesting feature of the story we have told is not only the way in which perceptions of professional interest change, but the noticeable tension between the *collective* interests of the profession whose peculiar relationship with the state has permitted it a degree of monopoly over the provision of health care, and the personal interests of the *individual* professional trying to make a satisfying living in an uncertain and changing climate. In Britain, as in some other countries, various state policies have helped to drive a wedge between the interests of the individual professional and that of the professional collective. This has been particularly prominent where quasi marketization of services such as health care and education has seriously weakened the power of professional groups. Thus in Britain, fundholding for GPS has created a space in which some GPS can ride with rather than resist public demand for alternative medicine by buying in the services of practitioners regarded as particularly useful and cost effective. In a number of countries broad definitions of medical practice have always permitted some doctors to practice some form of alternative medicine without their more orthodox peers having much recourse to either law or disciplinary procedures. If governments have no incentive to tighten up the law (and most seem to be going in the opposite direction) the medical profession is unlikely to be able to exercise any very tight control over what goes on in the consulting room.

At the same time, a political demand for tight control over public expenditure creates a climate in which the representatives of orthodox medicine may very reasonably entertain anxiety about their status *vis-à-vis* the state, fearing diversion of funds from the kinds of research and medicine which they practice themselves. As we saw in the British case there is enough state interest in the issue of cost effectiveness of alternative medicines to justify such anxiety. Easthope has likewise argued, in relation to Australia, that we need to look at the market for health in a situation where the Treasury is concerned to keep expenditure on health care down and increasing government attention is being paid to the idea of preventive rather than interventive medicine. If alternative medicine is perceived to be cheaper than biomedicine, it may begin to have attractions for those in government (Easthope 1993:299).

Official medical bodies have to make a decision as to whether to resist state endorsement of alternative medicine or whether to anticipate the issue by endorsing it themselves, and incorporating it into their own repertoires. The timing is not easy to decide. The BMA probably turned its views around just in time to avoid total embarrassment. In Sweden and Australia national medical associations have held out for longer. In France the collectivity has been in a securer position, but individual practitioners have chosen either way, some colluding in the prosecution of deviant colleagues and some practising alternative therapies themselves.

The crumbling of organized professional opposition to alternative medicines in Britain in the face of its public popularity calls into question straightforward notions of medical dominance and medical self-interest. That is, we cannot make sense of the relations between biomedicine and alternative medicine *without* the concepts of medical dominance and professional self-interest, but they do not adequately explain certain trains of events *on their own*. In particular, they are insufficient to account for the variety and shifts in medical attitudes that we have discussed in this chapter. Medical attitudes to alternative medicines need to be looked at in a wider political context. We learn less from looking at the orthodox medicine/alternative medicine dyad than we do from examining the orthodox medicine/alternative medicine/state triad. We examine this web of relationships and the way they shape policy in the following chapter.

CHAPTER 5

Government responses:
the refiguring of expertise

Theoretical approaches

The depth and range of intervention by the state in the social and economic life of a society varies across time and space. Nevertheless, a defining feature of all states is this potential to intervene, and through this intervention to determine the boundaries and rules of all other activity in a community. In communities with a well developed "Welfare State", the role of the state in the shaping of the health care market is paramount. This is particularly so in the United Kingdom, the National Health Service (NHS) being a state organization. This is not to say that all health care is provided by the state; we know that much care is dispensed in the informal sector and that increasing numbers of consumers seek care from the private and complementary medical sectors, arenas that do not usually receive state funding. Nevertheless, states have a part to play in setting the rules of the market and the regulation of activity in these sectors and may, in Europe, be required to extend regulative powers further as a result of European Union directives (Lannoye 1997).[1]

In this chapter we explore state intervention in health care, and examine the extent to which the state has endorsed or curtailed the development of a plural medical market. It is the tactics of government which delineate what is permissible in health terms and this chapter thus analyses the willingness of governments, particularly the British Government, to legislate on health matters and how this may have changed over time. It is possible to conceive that the state could support alternative medical groups in a number of ways, including state registration which protects the title of the practitioner, the funding of educational programmes, the granting of research funds, the inclusion in insurance schemes and, in the case of Britain, the inclusion of therapies in the state NHS.

However, such decisions are always made in the context of economic, political and ideological considerations and according to historical and geographical location. Specifically, the state has to maintain a relationship between itself, civil society and the economy and must balance the contradictory needs of consent (societal acceptance of its intervention) with constraint (the enhancement of societal stability through surveillance) and capitalism (see Hay 1996). Thus, changes in civil demands and the economy always necessitate changes to state structures. The recent revival of alternative medicine has coincided with changes to the way that the British State has organized its role in welfare provision. The post-war settlement saw a commitment to a universalistic and Keynesian welfare state (welfare capitalism), albeit one that at the time only provided *biomedicine* (with the exception of homoeopathy, delivered by biomedically qualified doctors) free at the point of delivery. This provision can be seen as the result of class compromise (Offe 1984) and was built on the commitment to active, interventionist government, social welfare provision and a dependence upon professional expertise (Hay 1996). Such provision allowed the state to regulate civil society, secure state legitimacy and contain social demands but inevitably imposed a heavy financial burden.

The inevitable contradiction between capitalist accumulation and societal legitimation (theorized by neo-Marxists as a legitimation crisis – see Habermas 1975) meant that such provision could not be sustained (Hay 1996) and necessitated structural changes to the boundaries of what constituted state intervention. This fiscal crises was, in Britain, translated via an ideological stance, exemplified by the New Right and Thatcherism, that questioned the support of monopolies and was committed to a shift in the balance of public and private provision of welfare services. Overall, we have seen a distancing from the commitment to full and prescriptive welfare provision to be replaced by a service arrangement that is flexible and responsive, which makes minimal demands upon the public purse yet facilitates consumerism and individual responsibility. In health care the response was to introduce internal markets and encourage the expansion of the private sector. More recently, this solution has lost public support and the Labour Government, ushered into power in 1997, has the task of responding to criticisms that welfare provision is under extended and retrenched but at the same time must provide a health care system within stringent financial limits. Thus, it is this wider context that inevitably underpins any decisions that might be taken with regard to alternative medicine. In the remainder of this chapter we review the empirical changes that have occurred.

Furthermore, there are a range of historical and geographical preconditions that shape the precise way in which various states privilege biomedicine and the means by which other forms of health care are disprivileged. Last (1990) has devised a typology of "national medical cultures" which is helpful here. He identifies the following models:

a) "Exclusive Systems", including:
   i)   The French Model; centralized state control. Unlicensed healers are illegal, non-biomedical healing is only permitted to registered doctors who are themselves largely employed as civil servants under close control of the state.
   ii) The (former) Soviet model; medicine itself has a low level of professional independence from the state, but either the state outlaws other kinds of healing or offers them no institutional space in which to develop (the public health care is based on biomedicine and private professional practice is not permitted).
   iii) The American model; free medical market regulated by state or federal licensing laws. The state has a policing role in seeing that practitioners do not practice what they are not licensed to practice.

b) "Tolerant systems", including:
   i)   The British model; non-biomedical healers are not outlawed, they are only forbidden to call themselves doctors. However they largely operate outside the state run system of health care.
   ii) The German model; non-biomedical healers of various kinds are licensed by the state as "heilpraktiker" if they can

pass an examination to show that they understand the law regulating medical practice, and can recognize a wide range of "notifiable" diseases.

c) "Integrative systems", including:

  i) The Indian and Chinese models; biomedicine is privileged but certain other systems of healing are recognized by the state and may receive some degree of state support. In India support is extended to Ayurvedic medicine and to homoeopathy, and in China, traditional Chinese medicine in various forms is integrated into the state run system of health care.

  ii) The "Third World model"; biomedicine enjoys legal privileges and some state support, but it is not strong enough in practice to secure any kind of monopoly in the overall system of health care.

This typology has its problems, but many of these spring from the fact that things are changing rapidly. Many of the systems that in terms of statutory position would fall into the exclusive category have *de facto* approached something more like the permissive British system, in as much as laws designed to outlaw non-biomedical practice are falling into desuetude or proving difficult to apply (although the arrest in 1996 of three non-medically qualified homoeopaths in Belgium, who had previously practised illegally (Gordon 1997a), suggest that this situation cannot be assumed). Increasingly, we find a distinction not just between legitimate biomedicine and illegitimate alternative medicine, but between legitimated therapies with state registration of some kind and those without (which remain tolerated or forbidden). A few concrete examples will illustrate the complexity of the situation.

For instance, while from some points of view the United States of America and Britain belong to different categories, there is a degree of convergence towards a situation where certain therapies are recognized and licensed. In Britain the granting of statutory regulation to the osteopaths and chiropractors has created a distinction between favoured and less favoured therapies. In the United States, alternative medicine has been controlled and limited by licensing laws (although these vary from state to state) and the Food and Drugs Administration has had the power to define which medicines are safe and legal. The federal government has also recently taken more interest with the directive from Congress for the National Institute of Health to open an office of Alternative Medicine and provide funds for research. In spite of much opposition to alternative therapies from the American Medical Association, at least 29 medical schools in the United States now have courses relating to alternative medicine (Pavek 1995).

In some states hybridity was built into the system from the start. South Africa could be described as having a fairly "tolerant" system until some quite stringent laws were passed in the 1970s effectively closing down the possibility of practising legally for alternative therapists not already in practice at the time. However, only a decade later in 1982, the South Africa Council for the Associated Health Service Professions was charged with the task of devising a way of defining and controlling the alternative therapies, and in 1985 it was empowered to open a register for practitioners (Pretorius 1993). However, this legislation effectively only controlled the kinds of therapies used mainly by whites and in urban areas. It has had little effect on the use of traditional healers by rural Africans, who for the most part do not have adequate access to biomedical facilities. From the point of view of rural Africans, South Africa looked much more like Last's "Third World model".

Another kind of complexity is exemplified in the case of the Netherlands. Since 1865, legitimate medical practice has been restricted to qualified doctors. However, a government committee was set up in 1970 occasioned by awareness that the Dutch public were very favourable to alternative medicine and were exerting considerable pressure for freedom to choose the therapy they wished to use. The Commission produced a report supportive of alternative medicine and a further commission was set up to investigate appropriate policies for this group of therapies. New legislation was drafted (the Individual Health Care Professions Act), which would legitimate the provision of medical treatment by practitioners of any therapy (with the exception of surgery and some other procedures which would still be performed by qualified doctors). However, this legislation was only adopted in draft form in 1993 (Menges 1994, Fulder 1996, Gordon 1997a). The interest in this example lies in the long gestation period of new legislation and that the Dutch system continued to be what Last would call an "exclusive" system but in practice was "tolerant".

From these examples we see that national medical cultures show complexity and contradictions and are liable to vary considerably over time. The general tendency has been in the direction of greater effective tolerance, particularly for those therapies that have standardized their training and defined a sphere of competence (see Ch. 3 for more details in this area). However, we do not wish to present an overly uniform picture (although further harmonization in the case of Europe is likely) and nor do we wish to suggest that government registration will necessarily signify availability in any state provided health care service.

In the United Kingdom, where common law prevails and anyone who designates him or herself as a healer can practice ("the tolerant framework"), it may appear that the government exhibits an indifference to the wider complexion of the medical services and indeed that the therapists themselves are not as concerned about their legal standing as in other countries. Nevertheless, perceived threats to the practice of complementary medicine (Cant & Sharma 1994, and see Ch. 3) and the increased use of complementary medicine by patients (see Ch. 2) have meant that common law alone has not been seen as sufficient protection for all parties.

However, as in most western states there exists a special relationship between the state and the orthodox medical profession, one that has supported an orthodox medical monopoly until recent years and has caused commentators to suggest that the medical profession is in fact an agent of the state (Navarro 1978, Doyal 1979) or in Foucault's understanding of governmentality (1979) that the medical profession *is* the state (Johnson 1996). Such a conceptualization does not see the state or the medical profession as separate entities, with separate histories, nor does it make any assumptions about the dominance or decline of the medical profession. Both the state and the medical profession are seen as part of a general process of regulation and involved in the "technologies of power". Both generate discourses and work together to define the possible parameters of governance of the population. The emergence of institutionalized expertise was, for Foucault, integral to governmentality, a novel capacity for government that uses knowledge, technologies, discourses and tactics to survey, regulate and normalize the population. Professionals, such as doctors, are then critical for the development and maintenance of this governing capacity. If we take on board such a reading, to what extent can the changes made in response to alternative medicine be viewed as part of the wider population governance? And, further, is it that greater support of alternative medicine is indicative of changes in the state–capital relationship?

Certainly, recent trends imply that complementary medicine may receive more favourable treatment by the government, evidenced in the UK by the passing of the Osteopaths (1993) and Chiropractic (1994) Acts and the increased provision of complementary medical services within the NHS (NAHAT 1993). Consequently our attention will be directed to an exploration of the shifts in state response. Such an analysis requires an examination of the "foreground" of the actual decision-making process and the "background" environment (Harrison et al. 1990), including the long rule by the Conservative Government and its encouragement of the private sector, its suspicion of monopolies and its commitment to consumer choice.

The concentration in this chapter is upon the British case and the experience of chiropractic, as this is one modality that has gained increased legitimacy in many countries. In our discussion we suggest that although there has been a pluralization of "legitimate" providers of health care and a restructuring of expertise, biomedicine itself has remained dominant.

First, however, we need to establish some ground rules for this analysis. Commonly, writers take the dominance of medicine as their starting point. This leads to the uncritical acceptance of the concept of "dominance" without attention to countervailing powers (Light 1996) and serves to direct our attention to shifts in medical power (proletarianization, etc.) as if it exists in a vacuum, thus often missing the importance of the dynamic relationship between professions, the government and the consumer (see also Coburn et al. 1997). In other words the medical profession, state/government and complementary medicine are viewed as separate entities, preconstituted and counterposed. It predicts a story of ruptures rather than negotiation and fails to acknowledge the interplay between these actors and indeed their commonalities. Research has, as Larkin (1996) argues, given separate and varied levels of attention to doctors, allied health professions and alternative practitioners rather than focussed on the frameworks which inextricably link and shape their individual histories (Larkin 1996: 45).

It also does not acknowledge the historical specificity of the concept of medical dominance itself (Light 1996). The boundaries of the health care market have always been contingent and are constantly in the process of negotiation. Thus, the boundaries of what is legitimate or dissident are always mediated by the relevant professional groups, the public and the politicians. The reader should keep in mind the dynamic and processual nature of these changes, even though we have, for the purposes of this book, divided up our subject matter.

Shifts in government intervention

To what extent has the government been involved in the provision and regulation of health care? In Britain we can, albeit very crudely, identify historical shifts in the level of activity by the government. Traditionally, we have seen a *laissez faire* approach to health care, the government seeming to prefer to be non-interventionist and non-proactive, the granting of Royal Charters being the extent of their interest (MacDonald 1995). However, the government became more open to involvement in the mid nineteenth century, and perhaps it is no surprise that this coincided with an increasing acceptance that knowledge could be scientific, unified and autonomous and that the state, experts and intellectuals could "legislate" in new areas (Bauman 1992). These ideological changes coincided then with the conterminous emergence of a monopoly for the medical profession, seen for a variety of reasons to be the "best" provider (partly because of their own professional project), and an increase in state power. The establishment of the NHS signifies the most important moment in this history, initiating state provision of health services and the establishment of the Welfare State. The medical profession was central to the allocation of health resources and thus the Welfare State has been dubbed the "Professional State" (Alaszewski 1996).

In more recent years, commentators (Ranade 1994, Allsop 1995, Klein 1995, Wall 1996) suggest that governments are attempting to reduce their involvement in welfare – the so called "rolling back of the state". Such a distancing from the provision of services is accompanied by the "New Right" ideology that stresses the need for competition, the curtailment of monopoly and the power of the consumer. This ideological stance has had practical ramifications for policy. For example, the most recent health care reforms (e.g. DOH 1989a, etc.) have provided for the establishment of an internal market which has included: competition with the contracting out of services; the empowerment of managers over other professional groups (Pollitt 1993); the curtailment of professional power (e.g. deregulation of optical services, DHSS 1984); the support of the private sector through encouragement of private health insurance (Calnan et al. 1993), the increase of private patients in the NHS and the greater flexibility for consultants to earn money in the private sector (Higgins 1988, Allsop 1995) and greater opportunities for choice and redress for the patient (see Patients Charter, DOH 1992). Moreover, the 1990 legislation created internal markets; so that the NHS was divided into purchasers and providers with much greater decentralization and more local determination of provision. The general practitioners (GPs) earned greater powers through these reforms (Allsop 1995) having the opportunity to deploy their budgets as they saw fit and this could include the purchase of complementary medical services (DOH 1991). Moreover, the reorientation of health service efforts to primary care (DOH 1989b) rather than the hospital also set a context where complementary medical services could be more important, especially as many therapists, e.g. homoeopaths, portray themselves as primary practitioners.

These shifts would appear to engender a conducive context for the development of a plural medical market – the encouragement of the private sector (Higgins 1988) and voluntary health services (Brenton 1985) effectively amount to the pluralization of health services. Nevertheless, it is interesting to note that all these reforms failed to explicitly mention complementary medical services and thus any advances that could be made had to be based on interpretation of the government's strategy and, as we shall show, have produced limited opportunities for integration of these services into the NHS (see Ch. 6).

Generally then, the British state appears to be more committed to a "hands off" approach that allows the patient to choose which-ever services they desire. At the same time, however, the state has a continued role in the regulation of health care services, to protect the patient from discreditable practitioners. Indeed, Klein (1995) depicts the latest health care reforms (DOH 1989b, etc.) as a shift from a *Welfare State* to a *Regulatory State*. And as Ranade argues, "the broad trend towards welfare pluralism is clear cut: the govern-ment as the main service provider is giving way to government by contract and regulation" (1994:151). Such a shift is further encour-aged by European Union intervention that requires common stand-ards across Europe and the harmonization of what is regulated and permissible. Thus, we can see a context for pluralism, one with an increased number of providers, but one where the providers have to perform according to certain regulative principles. These contextual changes provide another backdrop from which we can explore the extent to which practical policy has changed and indeed the extent to which this New Right ideology has been definitive.

The state, interest groups and health policy

How do we conceive of state/government activity? What prompts the state to become involved in an area of social and economic life? In particular, what is the catalyst behind health policy? Political science analysts of health policy tend to draw upon either *Marxist* analysis (Doyal 1979), seeing policy as constructed in the interests of capitalism and recognizing the importance of strategic elites, or *Pluralist* analysis (Alford 1975).[2] With the latter, the emphasis is upon the role of the interest groups upon public policy, rather than the unpersuaded work of political parties, and society is viewed as "open" with many interests that compete to influence government policy, larger groups having more influence. This rather simplistic picture has, of course, been criticized; the instance of the British Medical Association (BMA), in particular, has been used to show the exceptional influence of a relatively small group. Sociological per-spectives have similarly focused upon the importance of profes-sional activity (Freidson 1970) in the development of health services. In sum, there is an overarching recognition that certain groups have more power in health policy-making.

It is possible then to characterize the BMA as an "insider" group (Grant 1985), having the ear of government through its degree of respect, internal organization and contacts (Eckstein 1960). The important point is that "insider" status is not fixed and indeed where the government encouraged such relationships pre-1979, the Conservatives (1979–97) rejected corporatism and discouraged such influences upon policy. The policy process has always been about bidding, compromise, checks and balances and bargaining (even the creation of the NHS brought about gains and losses for the BMA), but the number of interests that jockey for position may become greater.

In this chapter we want to assess the relationship between the state and the various relevant interest groups and also how this may have changed. In particular, has the BMA lost its location as an insider group as a result of the entry of new groups and the government's disinclination to support monopolies more generally? How have other groups managed to gain support from the state and secure, even if temporararily, insider status? Before we explore this more fully, it is worth giving some brief attention to how and why the medical profession managed to achieve insider status.

The state and the medical profession: a special relationship?

In Britain, at least, the state has historically worked in favour of the orthodox medical profession. Although the passing of the Medical Act in 1858 was a hard won battle (Waddington 1984) and there is evidence to suggest that some doctors resisted close relations with the state (Honigsbaum 1979, MacDonald 1995), the implications were far reaching and favourable. Effectively the Act established that only certain practitioners could call themselves doctors, engage in self regulation, sue for fees and claim to treat certain categories of illness (Saks 1996). At this time the "medical profession"[3] was still engaged in a "territorial battle" (Abbott 1988) with other practitioners. Orthodoxy launched an attack on what it perceived to be quackery and with the support of the state was able to dominate the health care market in total through strategies of discreditation, elimination, limitation and subordination (Larkin 1983, Nicholls 1988, Willis 1989, etc.). In particular, the close relationship with the state was apparent in the passing of health legislation in the twentieth century, especially the establishment of the National Health Service, which only provided for the inclusion of the Royal Homoeopathic Hospitals under state funding. With the state provision of orthodox medicine, it was no surprise that consumers were attracted to health care that was free at the point of delivery rather than alternative medicine that was firmly ensconced in the private sector. In other words, this special relationship provided for a *medical model* of state health care, and the commitment to *allopathic* care for the general population.

It was not simply that orthodox medicine secured a monopoly but, importantly, that they became experts in the consultation of all health policy. After the First World War, doctors staffed the newly formed Ministry of Health (Larkin 1996), and medical representatives were seated on all consultative councils and advisory bodies (Kingdom 1990). As Klein argues, "the medical profession permeated the decision-making machinery of the NHS at every level and achieved an effective right of veto" (1995:49), and thus wielded enormous power over decisions such as which health issues would or could be discussed.

This long standing relationship between the medical profession and the state has meant that their interests have become intimately entwined, so much so that at times they are synonymous. During the hearing of the Osteopaths Bill (for state regulation), for instance, the BMA and the Kings Fund were important consultants.

However, there is evidence to suggest that this special relationship may be changing. Baggott (1995:44) suggests that whereas the BMA and Department of Health (DOH) used to have a bipartite relationship, the New Right have become suspicious of such a corporatist relationship. In particular, the latest health care reforms were introduced without the broad support of, and without consultation with the BMA, as Baggott outlines,

> although the BMA dropped its opposition to some government policies (e.g. fundholding) it remained highly critical of the impact of the internal market [and] . . . continued to protest that

it was not consulted on policy matters . . . One particular concern has been the short amount of time allowed for comments on consultative documents. For example it was reported in the medical press that the DOH requested comments from the BMA on a twenty page document (on the subject of clinical audit) within twenty-four hours (Baggott 1995:128).

In summary, the BMA, with its insider status, has held a characteristically powerful position and has been able to influence the government. However, this relationship appears to be changing and there is some evidence that the two groups have become increasingly estranged, the state becoming more suspicious of producer interest groups that obstruct the free play of the market.

This picture is not peculiar to the United Kingdom (Johnson et al. 1996). Whereas the majority of studies take the demise of medical dominance as their focus, without locating the wider contextual changes, there is evidence in this literature alone that biomedical professions have lost some of their powers, but not that medicine has declined as the dominant discourse. Generally, across Europe we have seen the proletarianization of the medical profession (e.g. in Spain see Rodriquez 1996) and the increased powers of other professionals (e.g. midwives in the Netherlands in the work of Van Teijlingen & Van der Hulst 1996). Willis's (1989) work in Australia similarly suggests that the state has become less willing to give *carte blanche* support for the medical profession and this is illustrated by its support for statutory regulation of other groups of practitioners. In the United States, licensing laws have been granted for alternative practitioners, although these vary from state to state (Sale 1995), and there is evidence that the power of the orthodox medical profession has been curtailed.

The state and complementary medicine: a changing relationship?

If the relationship between the orthodox medical profession and the state has been exclusive, where does this leave complementary medicine? We could conceive of complementary medical practice as entirely marginal to the interests of the state and history would

suggest we should draw the same conclusion. The exclusion of complementary medicines from the NHS in 1948 was disastrous for their
practice, and it is at this time that we see the decline in number of
practitioners.[4] There are also instances of damaging legislation such
as that which banned the use of the comfrey herb (Whitelegg 1996).
Notwithstanding such evidence, it is possible to locate occasions
when the government has acted in a more favourable way –
although these are few and far between – for example, the BMA was
not able to prevent the entry of spiritual healers to the NHS in the
1950s and 1960s (Inglis 1980). The last decade has seen increasing
instances of supportive action by the state, partly generated no
doubt by the increased interest in complementary medicine by consumers, so that it is possible to ask whether the orthodox medical
profession–state relationship has run its course, to be replaced by a
more pluralistic phase.

Larkin (1983) suggests that practitioner groups have historically
attempted to break the state–physician alliance by relying on three
strategies: first, through public support, secondly, by securing a
Royal Charter and inclusion under the Companies Act, or thirdly,
by state registration.[5] Within complementary medicine it is the first
strategy that has been used most widely until recent times. Indeed,
the twentieth century has largely been characterized by the
thwarted attempts of complementary medical groups to gain recognition from the state. At a time when the registration of midwives
(1902), nurses (1919), dentists (1921) were successful, albeit placing
them in subordinate positions in the medical division of labour, the
complementary therapists met with no success. The osteopaths and
herbalists made several submissions during the 1920s and 1930s
(Larkin 1996), but were dismissed with incredulity. Larkin shows
that this dismissal was the product of the state's use of the medical
profession as advisors. The herbalists for example,

> discovered that what they regarded as their correspondence
> with the Minister of Health in fact was being passed onto the
> General Medical Council (GMC) to advise the Ministry of
> Health, and in turn being relayed to the pharmacy profession to
> stimulate its opposition in addition to that of the medical profes-
> sion. (Larkin 1996:49)

The Osteopaths Bill also had numerous opponents including the BMA, GMC, Royal Colleges of Surgeons, the Royal College of Physicians and Medical Schools (Baer 1984b) and similarly, chiropractic had a failed attempt to be registered as a profession supplementary to medicine in 1975.

The 1980s and 1990s have been witness to a changing relationship between the state and complementary medicine in Britain. In 1989 the All Party Group for Complementary and Alternative Medicine was set up with the remit to prevent damaging legislation and to promote the use of complementary medicine within the NHS (PGACM 1993). A research study conducted for the Research Council of Complementary Medicine assessed the general degree of support for complementary medicine by Members of Parliament (RCCM 1991) and revealed high degrees of support for therapies to be included in the NHS especially osteopathy (74 per cent), acupuncture (62 per cent), chiropractic (50 per cent) and homoeopathy (53 per cent). Levels of support did, however, vary when controlled for party affiliation, Labour MPs being more supportive.

When we turn our attention to specific responses that have emanated from government we see there have been three policy initiatives that have had knock on effects for complementary medicine. In the first place, following the NHS reforms (1990) the then Junior Minister for Health, Steven Dorrell, was asked to clarify the position for complementary medicine. His statement confirmed that GP fundholders could use their budgets to purchase complementary medical services. A study by the Medical Care Research Unit in Sheffield (Thomas et al. 1995) has more recently assessed the use of this right and showed that referral rates were low, but that 39.5 per cent of GPs did provide access to some forms of complementary therapy for their NHS patients. Acupuncture, homoeopathy and osteopathy were the most popular choices.

Secondly, a number of statements have been issued regarding the criteria under which the government might contemplate the statutory registration of complementary medicine. The expected criteria were that the therapy should be based on a systematic body of knowledge, there should be voluntary registration in place that embraced an appropriate and enforceable code of conduct, the profession should exhibit unity and finally should have the support of the medical profession (HMSO 1987). Since that time we have seen the successful passing of the Osteopaths and Chiropractors Acts. The acupuncturists and homoeopaths were also, at the time of writing, in the process of preliminary discussions.

Thirdly, the NHS reforms have given the opportunity to re-orientate heath care services, in particular, a large number of Family Health Service Authorities (FHSAs) are using the "health promotion clinic" budget to support complementary therapists. A study undertaken by NAHAT in 1992 estimated that £1m of the NHS budget, a small sum in the light of the overall expenditure on health, had been spent on complementary medical services (NAHAT 1993).

Generally then, the Conservative Government made some positive overtures to the complementary therapists. The Labour Government, elected in 1997, had published a discussion document about complementary medical services prior to election which suggested stronger commitment, with calls for strategic policy to integrate osteopathy, chiropractic and acupuncture into the NHS (Primarolo 1992) and the establishment of an Office for Complementary Medicine through the Department of Health.

This shift in attitude towards complementary medicine is not peculiar to Britain alone and in many instances the UK has in fact lagged behind other countries. In the United States, some individual states have allowed certain groups (e.g. trained acupuncturists) to practice independently of the medical profession (Saks 1995). Chiropractic has achieved state regulation in all American states since 1974 although the realities of this regulation vary, in some states for instance, the medical profession retains control and has dictated the content of chiropractic education. Chiropractic has also attracted state regulation in Australia (Willis 1989), Canada (Coburn & Biggs 1986) and New Zealand. In Europe we see two diametrically opposed views for complementary medicine. The first is based on the premiss that only the medical profession is legally able to provide such practice, e.g. France, Belgium and Luxembourg, although illegal practice is often ignored in practice. The second is more open, the various states allowing practitioners freedom and in some cases endorsing their therapy. For example, in Switzerland, Norway, Finland and Sweden (see Pedersen 1990) statutory legislation for chiropractic has been passed. Since 1993 in the Netherlands, a law has allowed anyone to practice medicine but does list some reserved practices (Lannoye 1997), and in Germany, as discussed earlier, the freedom to practice health care has existed since 1873 and the profession of "heilpraktiker" has been recognized since 1939, allowing other practitioners (not necessarily medically qualified) to offer alternative therapies if they have undertaken a common examination.

How might we explain this intensified interest? One explanation must hinge on economic factors. There has been increasing global concern about the escalating costs of medical care, not only the rise of health budgets (at a time when the range and application of health care becomes increasingly wide) but also the time and money lost on intractable conditions, those not amenable to cure by the medical profession. It was in the light of such concerns that the Back Pain Group was inaugurated in 1976 in the UK (Baer 1984b) with the remit to assess other services that might be more cost effective. With such an explanation we might expect to see the increase of research funds to assess the effectiveness of approaches and that the therapies be ensconced within the private sector. Secondly, it is possible that the development of other therapies fill a gap in supply of medical personnel and certainly this is the explanation given by Baer (1984a) for the inclusion of chiropractic in the United States. This interpretation would appear to lack the same explanatory power in the United Kingdom. Thirdly, it could be that the government is responding to popular opinion (the therapists and their patients have been involved in very well orchestrated lobbying, e.g. letter writing campaign by chiropractic patients). It is no surprise that the softening of the government's approach coincided with the publication of numerous polls that showed the public support for and use of other services. Other strategic elites may also have been influential, the Royal family being the most public supporter of complementary medicine[6] in the UK, and certainly the medical profession has become more open to the development of complementary medicine. We explore the explanatory power of these factors and the extent to which the support of a plural health market can be witnessed in a detailed case study of chiropractic in the UK. We detail the steps that were required by the group themselves, the response of the medical profession and the actual rewards of state support.

The chiropractors: a case study

After over 60 years of campaigning, 1993 saw the passing of the Osteopaths Act and 1994 saw the chiropractors receive similar state regulation. Yet, it was only in 1991 that Baer concluded his study of these two therapeutic modalities with, "in the foreseeable future the Conservative government is unlikely to grant statutory recognition ... particularly as independent practitioners" (Baer 1991:45). What produced this apparent sea change in the government's approach to complementary medicine?

Origins and history of chiropractic

Chiropractic is the third largest primary health care profession in the world after medicine and dentistry (Wardwell 1992). In the UK, despite the small number of members (900 in March 1994), it is the most widely used complementary approach after osteopathy and it has been estimated that chiropractors see 75,000 patients a week (HMSO 1994a). Chiropractic was actually "discovered" in 1895 by Daniel David Palmer who had experimented with the manipulation of vertebrae, and the technique was imported to the UK in the early 1920s.

There has also been an on-going division within chiropractic relating to scope of practice. A consensus exists that chiropractic has the ability to resolve musculo-skeletal conditions – "type M" problems. However, it was also believed, by the early chiropractors and a body of the profession today, that energy from the brain is transmitted by the spinal cord and then to every organ in the body. Any abnormal function in organs has also been associated with subluxations at specific levels of the spine and so can be alleviated by manipulation. Thus, chiropractic has been said to alleviate "type O" (organic) problems.

Competition from the osteopaths, who put a bill before parliament in 1925, prompted the then 19 British chiropractors to form the British Chiropractic Association (BCA). The coming of the NHS proved problematic for chiropractic because they were no longer covered by insurance and consequently the profession went into decline. As a result of this descent in popularity the BCA decided to shift to a broader range of technical chiropractic methods, rejecting their previous adherence to the "straight" technique (Copeland Griffiths 1991). In 1965, the Anglo-European College of Chiropractic (AECC) opened its doors prepared to teach these various methods of chiropractic and significantly, in May 1988, the Council for National and Academic Awards (CNAA) accredited the course, making the AECC the first college of complementary or alternative medicine in Europe to offer a validated degree.

The operation of common law in the UK has meant that the BCA could not prevent other schools and practitioners setting up practice. There are currently two other forms of chiropractic in the UK (McTimoneys and McTimoney Corleys) which both conform to a "straight" form of practice with concentration on a single technique of manipulation.

This description is by way of background to the latest successful claim made by chiropractic to gain state regulation. A review of the BCA newsletters reveals that it was during 1988 that debates about regulation were renewed (an earlier submission had been made to the Professions Supplementary to Medicine in 1975 but had been rejected) because the BCA committee were anxious to police the profession:

> We need a protected title, every Tom, Dick and Harry can come under our banner, I mean ten years ago there wasn't any McTimoney, if we had had regulation then ... well we didn't, and its not going to be as easy now, because we have to unify with them ... we want to come in line with other recognized bodies so that we can police the profession and get basic standards. (Cant & Sharma 1994)

Making ready for registration

Following the regulation criteria set down by the government in 1987, it was recognized that to even begin a regulation campaign the three groups of chiropractors needed to come together and agree about standards. This was not going to be an easy task; for years the BCA membership had berated the McTimoneys and indeed wanted state regulation simply to get rid of this competition. Despite their differences the groups came together, convened a steering group (later a limited company) and worked very well together constituting, in effect, an umbrella body to represent the profession.

Unification was only part of the project to make themselves acceptable to the state. The preparations also included being able to prove they had a legitimate and scientific approach. This requirement has not been peculiar to Britain, indeed there have been international attempts to de-emphasize the more controversial elements of their treatment and secure a scientific paradigm to underpin their techniques (Coburn 1991). In other words, chiropractic has developed into a musculo-skeletal speciality. This is the way that the BCA portray themselves in their public relations literature:

> The zealous and unsupportable assertion of many chiropractors was that vertebral subluxation influencing the nervous system was the source of all or most of disease. This is as historical as the then current medical technique, bloodletting with the leech. This skeleton in the cupboard, rattled by a fringe movement of extremists as exist in any profession, has sometimes been the barrier to understanding and co-operation between the chiropractor and medical profession ... no responsible chiropractor today claims to cure organic disease through adjustment of the spine (BCA 1993).

Moreover, the BCA has also consciously aligned chiropractic to established scientific theory. As one member of the BCA stated;

> The biggest obstacle to increasing the therapy's potential is having an adequate knowledge base to fit to your hypotheses. I mean with the greatest respect to the homoeopaths their model is flawed, our model is based on standard orthopaedic principles and biomedical principles, so it is not our model – it's somebody else's that has been validated.

> (Interviewer) So you borrowed a model?

> Stolen basically ... we know we are empirically correct and now we have the science to prove it, the reason other therapies hate science is that they know they are correct but can't prove it. We are lucky that our empirical results are being supported by theory.

In other words, the chiropractors have linked themselves to the established medical paradigm. As in other countries, the development of chiropractic has been characterized by a *public* narrowing of practice and philosophy and the adoption of the scientific paradigm.

The medical profession – a steel fist in a velvet glove?

Until recently, as we discussed Chapter 4, the attitude of the medical profession towards complementary medicine in general has been unfavourable. This has taken the form of attempts to discredit the therapies as quackery. For example, an editorial in the *British Medical Journal* in 1983, described alternative medicine as a "phoney, pseudo scientific construction" and in the 1986 BMA report, chiropractic was described as follows:

> chiropractic . . . stem(s) from particular beliefs about the nature and causation of disease . . . These systems are incompatible with the corpus of scientific knowledge, and must be rejected by anyone who accepts the validity of the latter. (BMA 1986: 35)

An uproar followed the publication of the BMA report and this may have served to temper the reactions of the medical profession as the discreditation model had been shown to lack strength. The latest BMA report (1993) is certainly more favourable. In response to "discrete clinical disciplines" (such as homoeopathy and chiropractic) the report does not cast judgement about their efficacy but suggests that they should be subject to statutory regulation so as to ensure high standards and training and that medical science should be included in a core curriculum. There is a recognition that orthodox practitioners' training may be insufficient in these areas and that general practitioners and complementary therapists should work together.

While we have shown that the attitude of the medical profession has been changing, the BCA representative suggested that the medical profession had to be wooed by the chiropractors.

> We deliberately did not go straight and officially to the medical profession, because I think had we done that we would have run

into opposition because if it had gone to a committee there would have bound to have been someone or several on the committee who would have been opposed and would have stopped it moving forward . . . it was important not to get a "no" answer, you have to be non-confrontational. I have acted like this for our profession.

It was thus decided that the best thing was to win the medical profession round in more relaxed and informal circumstances . . . those of a dinner party:

> I had this idea, because the Prince of Wales had got people together from the medical profession before in a dinner party situation, that this was the way we could do it. Fortunately I knew X who had arranged previous dinner parties and he agreed to help, so we invited key people and the Kings Fund, and they all came. This was after the MRC trial and it was pretty clear that they supported us . . . After this the Department of Health decided that we appeared to have the support of the medical profession.

To summarize then, the attitude of the medical profession has undergone significant change and it appears that their support has been secured. This was not an easy or straightforward task but required extensive networking and was dependent to some degree upon the energy and persistence of the chair of the steering group and positive scientific results. Acceptance by the medical profession has meant compromise. Chiropractic has portrayed itself as a specialist and fitted into a gap in the medical market (back pain), an area in which the medical profession has had little success.

State registration and its provisions

The Chiropractors Bill was passed easily in 1994 and makes the provision for regulation, high standards of education and protection of the title of chiropractor, in the name of safeguarding the patient:

> There is great potential to do harm in untrained hands, to do a great deal of harm. The manipulation of necks and backs could be lethal without the proper degree of skill . . . equally importantly, serious underlying conditions for example, cancer, can

present symptoms very similar to back pain and the untrained manipulator may pursue in treatment (HMSO 1994b:1169).

The provision for a general council which maintains a statutory register and four committees responsible for education, complaints, health and professional conduct means that there are similarities with the 1858 Medical Act (except that there are provisions made for continuing education of members on the register and the disciplinary powers are more stringent than those of the General Medical Council).

In essence, this regulation provides for a *state supported profession in the private sector.* Moreover, a monopoly was not granted, rather it was clearly stated that other groups could practice chiropractic:

> The Bill protect(s) the title chiropractor ... and makes it a criminal offence for other than a registered practitioner to call himself by that name. I know that provision interests many related professions. I confirm that it is not intended to prevent other professions ... from using chiropractic techniques in the course of their treatment and from telling their patients that they are using such techniques (HMSO 1994b:1169),

and certainly there is nothing in the law to stop practitioners calling themselves a "bonesetter", for example, and practising chiropractic techniques.

What explanations can be provided for this statutory support? First, the issue of cost was certainly raised in the parliamentary debate:

> 310,000 people in the United Kingdom are off work each day with back pain. That costs the country more than £3 billion a year in lost production. Disability from lower back pain is increasing faster than any other form of disability (HMSO 1994b:1184),

and references were made to the Medical Research Council (MRC) report which compared the outcomes of chiropractic treatment with outpatient hospital treatment and concluded:

> For patients with low back pain in whom manipulation is not contraindicated chiropractic almost certainly confers worth-

while, long-term benefit in comparison with hospital outpatient management (Meade et al. 1990).

The government sponsorship was limited only to registration and was not concerned to extend any financial commitments and there were certainly no plans to provide blanket funding for chiropractic:

> The overwhelming majority of chiropractors practise in the private sector and that position is unlikely to alter even if the Bill succeeds (HMSO 1994b: 1176).

Nor was there provision for educational grants. So, while it was hoped the Bill would increase collaboration with orthodoxy there was no discussion of bringing chiropractic into the NHS. Rather, there was a direct linkage of chiropractic practice to the private sector,

> I hope the Bill will encourage more private insurers to cover chiropractic treatment, because they will judge it more cost effective than orthodox medical treatment (HMSO 1994b: 1181).

However, at a practical level, there are only a small number of chiropractors (900 at our last count) who are not dispersed evenly throughout the country. Thus, state regulation has not made the service more available to the public despite the arguments about the clinical and cost effectiveness of the approach.

Secondly, the incorporation of chiropractic has not challenged the current direction of health care. Chiropractic, as in other parts of the world, has taken on board a narrower definition of practice. Whereas state regulation may encourage a more favourable attitude on the part of purchasing GPs, the funding and health care system have not altered. Thus, chiropractors who want to take state patients will be dependant upon the GP as a gatekeeper. As such they will, in the final analysis, be subject to the attitudes of individual GPs and will be employed in a delegated role, with patients and problems defined by the GP. Stacey (1994) has warned that the advantages and disadvantages of state registration balance out differently for each therapy but that on the whole the price of state registration has been subordination to biomedicine. The disadvantages will, in the long run, depend on the extent to which each therapy sees its position in relation to biomedicine. Those that see themselves as truly complementary will have fewer problems. For others, registration may restrict the way they practice and only afford them a small space in the market and provide little more than boundary definition. Thus, by specializing, the chiropractors, like the dentists, have been bestowed a "part" of the body but, in the final analysis, may not have autonomy and control over this area. We see then that the state has been involved in the refiguring of expertise but without a radical change in the complexion of the health services.

Finally, the impact of public opinion and the more favourable attitude of the BMA were important contextual changes that must account partly for the more favourable attitude of the government. The chiropractors engaged their supporters in a massive letter writing campaign to MPs that heightened the awareness of the therapy. This, of course, occurred under a Conservative Government, who, as we have seen, were less influenced by professional advice and more by the mandate from the public and at a time of broader crisis for universalistic welfare provision.

Conclusions

The preceding discussion points to a number of shifts in governmental responses to complementary medicine, particularly changes to the content of medical care and context in which policy decisions are made. Historically, health care provision could be depicted as plural, simply by virtue of the inattention of the government. This shifted in the nineteenth century with a state–physician alliance, to monopolistic control by orthodox medicine, and more recently we have seen a refiguring of expertise. These changes are not peculiar to Britain and seem to have occurred even in countries with very different systems of government, partly, of course, because they have been consumer led. How pervasive are these changes and what are the implications for complementary medicine, the medical profession, and the intervention of the state in health matters?

Paradoxically, an ideology that supports the rolling back of the state coexists with a situation where governments are passing legislation to regulate therapies. This regulation has often tended to curtail practice and bring it in line with more medical definitions of the therapy. At the same time the increased state jurisdiction has not been activated by the orthodox medical profession alone, rather the state has taken account of public demand (it has had to pursue policies that society demands) and broader economic decisions relating to cost curtailment. However, the influence of an ideological commitment to neoclassical economics does not suffice in our explanation of these changes. We showed at the beginning of this chapter that state intervention is also propelled by the need to constrain and regulate the population. Therefore, the changes in the government's response should be seen as the product of the need to balance public demand with economic constraint and the prerequisite that there be social stability. Drawing on the contradictions of capitalism (specifically the need to curtail costs) and upon Foucault's concept of governmentality, we suggest that we are witnessing the restructuring of expertise. To reiterate, in Foucault's conception, the state and the medical profession are not separate entities but rather are intimately entwined, thus the professionalization of medicine cannot simply be explained by the success of its occupational strategies but rather as the institutionalization of expertise that is crucial to governmentality – the regulation and surveillance and normalization of populations. (Of course these surveillance functions can operate without state recognition or regulation if the holistic function increases knowledge about the individual patient and encourages self responsibility; see Lowenberg & Davis 1994, Braathen 1996.) The shift in the government's response can be understood as the refiguring of this governmentality. At the same time it is no coincidence that the organizational framework for this refiguring has been established in the private sector.

Practically, we have seen the refiguring of expertise as the government has intervened to ratify who is a legitimate provider. This is a significant change. Previously patients of chiropractors would choose their practitioner by word of mouth and recommendation. In other words, the charisma of the therapist (Cant 1996) and perceived success of the treatments provided by the practitioners would have been influential. Now we have a situation of the state identifying which practitioners may be viewed as "expert", based on training, credentials and internal organization. Thus, new criteria underpin the legitimacy of provider groups, and the clinical legitimacy as simply experienced by patient is less important. The state has stepped in to legislate where consumers did so before.

There has been a refiguring of exactly what types of expertise will attract state support. Orthodox medicine is no longer the only medical provider to receive sponsorship, indeed there has been some depreciation of the claims to expertise on behalf of the orthodox medical profession. Markets have not been freed, as neoclassical economists would have us believe, but restructured. The state has reduced direct provision but allowed the restructuring (albeit limited) of expertise in new ways, which has had some knock on effects for the jurisdiction of orthodox medicine and the relations between orthodox and complementary medicine. More broadly, as we have seen in Chapter 3, with the intervention of the European Union, there has been an "internationalization" of expertise in the context of a single market.

So, to reiterate, why has there been a need to refigure the expertise? Certainly there has been a loss of faith in orthodox medicine, and governments have needed to confront the problems of financial crisis and chronic illness. There has been a balancing of a number of contradictory demands, between those financial constraints of capitalism, the need to order and survey the population and yet also the need to respond to civil demands. As Johnson (1993) points out, the perception of the consumer has been incredibly important:

> Government initiated reform has, in these recent reforms, been securely linked with the political commitment to the "sovereign consumer". In the case of reform in the NHS, this translates into a shift of behaviour from the primary obligation of the sick to seek medical advice, as a means of social control, to a new set of obligations including the stress on prevention, the obligation to care for the self by adopting a healthy lifestyle ... The changes initiated in state-expert government structures are then, the product of new policy goals which include as part of the process, changing the way the citizen-subject normally relates to health care provision (Johnson 1993:149).

The passing of the osteopaths and chiropractors acts served to "normalize" their practice and legitimate their extended use. What we have seen, then, are changes to the boundaries of what is acceptable medical practice, a settlement that has tried to limit the demands upon the public purse and has rearticulated the state–profession relationship to create a new set of techniques and roles for the purposes of governmentality.

Why have only certain therapies, particularly, osteopathy and chiropractic, been endorsed in this way? In the first place, they do not significantly challenge orthodox medicine, indeed their acceptance has hinged on the therapies taking on board orthodox science and training (also see Ch. 3). However, it is possible to envisage a scenario in the future where other therapies may become more legitimate (certainly, the government in Britain and elsewhere has accepted the practice of other therapies and encouraged their use so long as practitioners are self regulated) especially those that emphasize healthy living and preventative medicine.

The current restructuring of expertise need not cost the government money, as the therapies are largely ensconced in the private sector. Thus the content of state funded health care remains unaffected, indeed in Australia there has been a strong resistance to including complementary practices under the Medicare[7] scheme in the fear that this will discourage those with higher incomes from paying themselves and will make the services more widely available (Easthope 1993). Nevertheless, the context of health policy-making has shifted, the influence of the medical profession and their status as insider groups being threatened in preference to other interest groups. The medical profession does retain high levels of authority in areas where technical advice is deemed necessary, e.g. the granting of research funds, and it is significant that complementary medicine has been highly unsuccessful in such bids for funding. Our attention has been largely directed towards the United Kingdom and in countries with different systems for funding health care there will be variations although, undoubtedly, all countries are experiencing the same pressures, i.e. limited funds and chronic health problems. Encouraging the inclusion of complementary medicine under private health care schemes may be one way forward, but even this strategy has problems considering that some patients tend to continue to use complementary and orthodox medical services simultaneously and therefore do not withdraw from the services provided by the state (see Ch. 2).

Overall, we have seen changes to the practices of government.

154

The government has responded to consumer demand, the need to cut costs, the failures of orthodox medicine and in addition, has extended its regulative agenda. Consequently, the developments have often been contradictory, on the one hand we see the support of groups but on the other they are insufficiently financed. The consequence has been a refiguring of expertise rather than a radical alteration to the system of health care delivery.

Notes

1. The latest document to be produced by the European Union calls upon the Commission to recognize what it calls "non conventional medicine", to engage in research, to harmonize regulations (including the establishment of standards) and calls upon each Member State to consider including certain therapies into their social security systems. The responses to the report were being considered at the time of writing.
2. Here pluralism is distinct from medical pluralism and refers to equality between groups.
3. We have used inverted commas here because the medical profession had not fully coalesced into a clearly defined group.
4. The number of chiropractors dwindled at this time see Gaucher-Peslherbe (1986).
5. Groups can of course be self regulated, have state-sanctioned self-regulation or be directly administered by the state. Our discussion related to state-sanctioned self-regulation.
6. The Royal family has always supported homoeopathy. Prince Charles has been involved in private talks with representatives of the main complementary therapies and Lady Diana (as she was then) gave her support to the Chiropractors' campaign for state support.
7. Medicare came into effect in 1984 and is based on the principle of universal coverage against costs of medical care.

CHAPTER 6

Collaboration between doctors and alternative therapists: integration or medical dominance?

In the previous two chapters we have argued that there has been a limited legitimation of some alternative therapies. This was brought about by a number of factors, an important one being the greater acceptability of some alternative modalities to the medical profession. In both northern Europe and North America there is even talk of an "integration" of orthodox and alternative medicine. There is certainly greater scope than before for doctors and alternative practitioners of certain kinds to work together, and in Britain much of this collaboration is taking place within the state funded health care system.

In this chapter we ask how far there can be genuine coexistence and indeed co-operation between orthodox and alternative practitioners without the former dominating and transforming the latter. Can the pluralization of health care which we have described develop into the parallel and independent existence of a number of diverse healing modes? Or will the impetus to "integration" simply lead to the incorporation of certain holistic healing modes into the biomedical clinic without any concession of authority by the latter?

Medical dominance revisited

At various points in the preceding chapters we have referred to debates about the nature of medical dominance and whether it has changed or even declined as a result of various kinds of challenges to biomedicine. Sociologists have raised the possibility of a demedicalization of society, or at any rate a deprofessionalization of doctors (Elston 1991). A number of issues have fuelled this interest. One has been the realization that whereas the doctor may appear extremely powerful in relation to both patients and to other workers in the context of the clinic, there are a number of more general factors which could modify the social power of the medical profession overall. In Britain, the subordination of clinicians to the close control of managers who oversee the working of an internal market in the NHS has been seen as leading to a "fractured" form of dominance, even if this has not involved the actual proletarianization of doctors (Samson 1995). Not all countries have had a powerful and highly organized profession in the first place, and in some countries doctors have been very much the foot soldiers of a state bureaucracy. In such circumstances one might expect the presence of non-biomedical forms of healing to have potentially important consequences for medical power. For example, with respect to medical pluralism in India (where both Ayurveda and homoeopathy are recognized and supported by the state) Roger Jeffery has argued that there has been an actual deprofessionalization of medicine; while individual doctors have a high status and income, they have as a group to compete with other indigenous forms of medicine that also have official recognition (Jeffery 1977). In general, they have been less protected by the state from market forces than in countries like Britain. As we have seen, even European countries vary considerably as to the nature of the relationship between medicine and the state, and the degree of privilege this affords the medical profession. It is important to remember that the privilege and protection offered to biomedicine by the state has not everywhere been of the same degree or nature.

But where western countries are concerned, debates about medical dominance also refer to challenges to the general moral and professional authority of doctors in society. The voice of the consumer has become more doubting of the doctor's wisdom, more uncertain of the benefits that biomedicine can deliver when it has become over-technological, more critical of its impersonal delivery, etc. (Gabe et al. 1994, Williams & Calnan 1996). Professions such as nursing and midwifery have sought greater autonomy from medical control (Witz 1994).

On the whole, there is general agreement that the dominance of medicine (however dented) is still a powerful fact (Gabe et al. 1994), but a product of this discussion has been that medical hegemony has been problematized and less taken for granted as an automatic feature of any contemporary society. Some would even say we need to move beyond simple binary oppositions such as medicalization/ demedicalization; the crucial shift is the new focus on lifestyle and individual responsibility for one's health, a focus that is shared by physicians and alternative practitioners alike (Lowenberg & Davis 1994). Others would remind us that even if the medical profession has lost ground, medicine as a form of organized knowledge has not lost its hold. As Frankenberg shows (responding to Jeffery 1977, cited above), if Indian doctors have ceded ground as a group, it is still the case that medical understandings provide an important contribution to a capitalist ideology which reinforces state power through its capacity to individualize sickness (Frankenberg 1981) and evade confrontation with the ways in which sickness is actually produced by a harsh class system. This insight is no less applicable to countries like Britain.

It is probably this ideological dominance (as much as anything else) which alternative practitioners wrestle with when they express fears of biomedical control. There has been some ambivalence as to whether the interests and integrity of alternative healing are best served by co-operation with doctors. There are fears that it may simply lead to a co-option of skills, compromising that which makes alternative therapy distinctively holistic. While the opportunity to reach more patients and to achieve greater security of practice may be welcomed, there are anxieties as to whether biomedicine and alternative therapies are really compatible in the last analysis. One homoeopath states:

> I can't help thinking that we are perhaps being naive in our approach to working within the NHS when we have so much to do in order to explore the interface between homoeopathy and allopathy, dominated as it is by chemical medicine. Working within the NHS is an experiment we need to be in control of (Ryan 1994).

If these fears are grounded then the wider acceptance of alternative medicine may lead to only a limited form of medical pluralism. In a truly pluralistic system of health care (considered here as an ideal type) the non-biomedical forms of healing would have independent and parallel forms of organization and the patients/consumers would choose the one that they regarded as most suitable for their condition or requirements. Collaboration between practitioners would be on equal terms; there might be mutual influence and accommodation, but no single form of knowledge or practice would dominate overall. We could envisage the relations between the various elements of such a system as mediated by markets (open commercial competition) or in terms of some kind of division of healing labour, some socially agreed notion of which forms of healing are suited to which kinds of illness or which kind of patient. History suggests that plural systems in this sense are indeed an ideal type. What happens in practice is that some systems are inevitably affected by the general power and authority of others, whether or not their practitioners work together in the same clinic.

Perhaps a good starting point for this chapter would be the expectation that what we find will lie somewhere between this ideal pluralism and a situation of total and static medical dominance. What must concern us is the dynamics of interaction, and the institutional forms that shape these dynamics. Furthermore, we should be wary of treating medical power as some kind of zero sum game in which power lost by doctors is necessarily gained by patients, by other kinds of healer, or anyone else in civil society. However, the potential for a shift in the social relations of health is one which does need to be addressed.

What does "integration" of biomedicine and alternative medicine mean?

Integrated medicine is a loosely used term of international currency that can refer to virtually any situation in which alternative and orthodox medical knowledges or practitioners interact beyond the level of simple impersonal referral. It can refer to the use of alternative medicines or therapeutic techniques by biomedical professionals, but more specifically it has been used to describe:

1) clinics where biomedical and alternative practitioners collaborate or work alongside each other in a variety of institutional

arrangements. At present such collaboration takes place mainly within the primary health care sector;

2) the integration of alternative medical knowledge into biomedical education.

In this chapter we shall discuss these two types of "integration", attending to their effects on the social relations of health, and specifically to issues of empowerment. The evidence is mainly from Britain and Scandinavia. This is not to say that such experiments have not taken place elsewhere (there have been plenty in the USA – see Mattson 1982) but there appears to be a shortage of accessible empirical accounts of such ventures.

In Britain, such integration has started off at a very local level, often at the initiative of a particular medical doctor who has seen possibilities for the employment of a complementary therapist in a fundholding practice. A survey commissioned by the Department of Health found that 39.5 per cent of GPs were providing access to some kind of complementary therapy for their patients (Thomas et al. 1995). Pietroni (1992) lists the institutional arrangements through which complementary medicine might be integrated into general practice in Britain, and a recent document produced by the Foundation for Integrated Medicine (Foundation for Integrated Medicine 1997) provides a summary of the various ways in which complementary medicine is currently being delivered through the NHS at both primary and secondary levels. This integration has happened piecemeal, ahead of any urging on the part of either the organized voice of the medical profession or the government, and it had begun well before the publication of the 1993 BMA report with its more favourable approach to complementary medicine. On the whole such schemes have been favourably evaluated by the practitioners involved, although they often convey the need for clearer protocols for referral and communication among practitioners (e.g. Emanuel et al. 1996, Richardson 1996).

Nevertheless, local health authority managers have tended to argue that any integration of complementary therapies at a more general level (i.e. as a matter of policy) must be preceded by efforts to identify the ways in which complementary therapies can be demonstrated to be effective, to clarify good practice and to achieve a proper definition of responsibilities and competences. Thus the

West Yorkshire Health Authority (with support from the National Association of Health Authorities and Trusts) hosted a conference on complementary therapies in the NHS entitled "Added Value", at which the prevalence of and demand for complementary therapies was discussed, as well as the criteria by which such therapies should be evaluated (West Yorkshire Health Authority 1994). Some authorities have simply attempted to establish what the supply and demand for complementary therapies is like in their area in advance of developing regional policies as regards purchasing (e.g. Emslie et al. 1996).

In theory, the organization of therapeutic responsibility in the NHS should be straightforward enough. Under established BMA guidelines the GP retains overall clinical responsibility for the patient, but may *refer* a patient to a hospital specialist for the duration of some episode which requires specialist skills. Or the GP may delegate the carrying out of a particular treatment procedure to, e.g. a physiotherapist or a practice nurse. Whereas the term "referral" is regularly used by both doctors and others to describe the various processes by which a GP sends patients to a named complementary practitioner, there is some ambiguity as to whether the relations of complementary therapist and doctor should be modelled on those of the relationship between a (subordinate) practice nurse and a (dominant) GP or whether they are not more like the relationship between a hospital specialist and a generalist family doctor. Or perhaps they should be seen as representing a quite different structure of co-operation from either of these familiar models (BMA 1993:145)?

"Integrated" clinics and health centres: power and communication at the micro-level

When a GP and a complementary therapist collaborate in the treatment of a patient (regardless of how this co-operation is organized) communication is required between professionals whose healing practices may assume very different knowledge bases and who are used to different kinds of patient/practitioner relationship. This can be an issue in any kind of inter-professional collaboration, even that which occurs among alternative therapists themselves (see

English-Lueck 1990:25). There is also the possibility that they may come from different cultural and social class backgrounds, as Borchgrevink notes is the case in Norway (Borchgrevink 1994), although this has not been identified as an issue in Britain. A further complication may be ambiguity as to professional status in a context where such distinctions have traditionally been given much weight. Carol Moore, an acupuncturist employed in a GP practice in England notes uncertainty as to how much she ought to be paid, since her qualifications and status had no obvious equivalent in the existing NHS structure (Moore 1995:25).

Summarizing a study of the Marylebone Centre in London (a well established "integrated" clinic, founded in 1987), Peter Reason identifies some of the issues regarding knowledge and power that emerge when a group of GPs and complementary practitioners work together in the same practice. The Marylebone Centre was founded with the intention that relations between the doctors and the complementary therapists should not be hierarchical but based on mutual respect and learning. But this egalitarian ethos did not prevent the complementary practitioners from feeling disempowered on occasion. Disagreements over specific patients suggested covert conflicts as to what the clinic was really about. Reason suggests that such hidden conflicts will be difficult to resolve unless the practitioners of different kinds of healing develop some common framework of ideas (Reason 1991).

At first the Marylebone GPs met patients on arrival to discuss the therapeutic possibilities available. But this excluded the complementary practitioners from the initial session and created a situation where the patient depended on the GP to tell them what was good for them (Reason 1991:145). On the other hand when, to correct this situation, the group experimented with sessions in which patient could discuss problems with GP and complementary practitioners together, the latter felt unsure how much they could claim for their own therapy, and how far they could claim anything without seeming to criticize what the GP had already done for the patient. There were also issues about developing common languages to mediate the technical vocabularies of different disciplines when communicating about patients (Peters 1994). "Energy" for example proved common to the practitioners' therapeutic vocabularies, but could be both a bridge and a source of obfuscation:

Energy is a mystery word and perhaps, once the word *has* been deconstructed and accepted as abstract and subjective, it can be used as such in a working group. Still, a group trying to develop a common clinical language may find, as ours has, that careless use of the energy metaphor is a source of confusion; a noun which obstructs the search for necessary adjectives. For the sake of its own development, our interprofessional group had to confront such mystification, and risk desecrating a comfortably shared but unexamined energy myth. The process of exploring one's own and others' subjectivity is not comfortable; even less where pet beliefs have to be overthrown (Peters 1994:188).

In a study of a Danish Centre for Integrated Medicine, Jette Jul Nielsen has noted that the problem of a clinical metalanguage was in practice resolved by the use of metaphors, such as the body consisting of many "layers" or structural levels of symptomology. These metaphors were enabling in that they facilitated communication between professionals and across therapeutic traditions (biomedical and alternative). But they could only perform this function at a rather superficial level. For instance, the *layer* metaphors were used by different healers who far from agreed on the order of the layers – i.e. health problems. Nielsen suggests that this superficiality of communication was one reason why the centre foundered as a venture:

> The power of the metaphors combined with the impression they gave of agreement had the effect that conflicts between the views of the healers were not taken up in discussions before disagreements apparently were too severe to be overcome (Nielsen 1993:171).

In some situations this ambiguity is either not recognized explicitly, or is resolved in favour of biomedical language. Carol Moore, an acupuncturist, describes how in written reports on GP patients she felt constrained to use biomedical langauge to describe their symptoms and progress. This meant that some subjective factors, which had no place in conventional biomedical reporting, could not find their way into reports. In some cases the GP would suggest termination of acupuncture treatment if the symptoms defined as problematic from the medical point of view had not ameliorated, even though the patient was starting to "feel" better. Interestingly, patients themselves do not seem to have found difficulty in operating with two languages, using different terms to describe their experiences to acupuncturist and to GP (Moore 1995:24).

Communication is likely to be a problem in any multidisciplinary group; Kettle notes that in the Hoxton Health Group – a London project funded partly by the NHS and partly from other kinds of government and charitable funding – "tutorials in anatomy and physiology were provided and a joint diagnostic questionnaire developed" to overcome problems created by the lack of a common technical language (Kettle 1993:150). In this case it was not biomedicine that was emerging as the dominant cognitive model (the Hoxton on-site team consisted of complementary practitioners only) but acupuncture. At Warwick House, an integrated clinic in Somerset, this problem was addressed through discussion sessions about each other's knowledge bases and modes of practice, also from mutual observation sessions (Paterson & Peacock 1995).

An issue that emerged early on at Warwick House was the pattern of GP referral. Patients could either refer themselves or be referred by the GP to one of a group of complementary practitioners who practised on the premises. If GPs are still the gate keepers so far as the majority of patients are concerned, then their knowledge and perception of what complementary therapies can do (and which one is appropriate for a particular case) will be crucial. At Warwick House complementary practitioners felt more satisfied with the pattern of referrals once GPs had increased their understanding of the specific therapies and started to send a wider range of cases to them. Referrals became more personal as GPs came to know more about the particular complementary practitioners in the Centre. However, here both GPs and complementary practitioners felt that they wanted more opportunities to learn about each other's knowledge and practice than pressures of time allowed. Inappropriate GP referral was also cited as a problem for complementary practitioners at Phoenix, a multi-disciplinary practice organized on a rather similar model to Warwick House (Reason 1995), and was also seen as a problem at the Wells Park practice described by Budd et al. (1990).

Mutual learning is not just an issue of personal development, but affects practice very directly. In a Liverpool project funded by the NHS complementary practitioners practised in separate premises, seeing patients referred to them by local GPs. Here the therapists felt that the GPs were inclined to send mainly "heartsink" cases. Furthermore, the GPs had no close co-operative contact with the therapists working in the Centre, so were not in a position to observe what the therapies could do. Presumably it was equally difficult for complementary practitioners to learn more about GP outlook and practice. However the feeling on the part of the therapists that they were "under pressure for results" did not favour such mutual learning (Donnelly 1995).

To summarize, integrated clinics characteristically employ those who are highly committed to joint working yet even then there are practical problems of communication. These are partly the product of different professional vocabularies but relate also to taken for granted assumptions about the proper role and place of complementary medicine. These problems are not insurmountable but take time to resolve, a resource not abundantly available in public health care settings.

Primary health care and "dialogue groups" in the community

In some European countries experiments have taken place at the level of the locality rather than the clinic. "Dialogue groups" consist of meetings of GPs and alternative practitioners to explore each other's therapeutic models, analogous to groups that have been set up in some developing countries to facilitate co-operation and mutual understanding between doctors and traditional healers, such as the training project in Puerto Rico which brought together spiritist-healers and various medical personnel (nurses, psychiatrists, clinical psychologists, etc.) (Koss 1980). The group facilitated by Norwegian anthropologist Vigdis Christie (Christie 1991) started out with cautious mutual curiosity but eventually led to referrals and collaboration over treatment. The group managed to discover what they had in common as well as what was peculiar to particular therapies.

Discussing a comparable experiment in the Netherlands, Visser (1991) points out that such projects only create useful dialogue and collaboration among those already well disposed to each other. Those GPs who are antagonistic to alternative therapies are unlikely to get involved or to learn much if they do. In this study, funded by the Dutch government, a group of GPs and alternative practitioners undertook to exchange information on patients and met to discuss different therapies with reference to patients who had been receiving alternative treatment. After two-and-a-half years GPs had changed their attitudes and practices very little. The alternative therapists, however, had expected more of the collaboration and were less satisfied with the experiment (probably they had expected to get more referrals as a result). In this case the paradigmatic distance between the GPs and alternative practitioners ought not to have been great – the project only drew upon therapists who had a medical training or were physiotherapists. It would seem that while there had been no perceived conflict in advice or treatments given by GPs and alternative therapists, and while the volume of intercommunication had been quite high during the lifespan of the project, GPs had been somewhat less inclined to share information with therapists than vice versa; for instance, they were less likely to report to the therapist when they changed the patient's medication (Visser 1997).

If there is any general lesson to be drawn from all this it is probably that, as Visser points out, for integration to have positive results all parties must perceive some positive gain (not necessarily material gain, and not necessarily the same for each side). The potential gains for independent practitioners working in the private market are very general – they might expect more referrals, access to diagnostic facilities, prestige and status from working with GPs. For GPs, operating from the security of the biomedical clinic, the potential gains must be more specific – a way of dealing with "heartsink" or "fat envelope" patients, or a way of dealing with patients with intractable symptoms such as back pain. Each party will see collaboration as solving problems of different types and scale.

At the micro-level, therefore, the effects of medical dominance are institutional – that is, they are not automatically neutralized by whatever respect the individual GPs may have for complementary therapies or other competences. The complementary therapists are at risk of feeling disempowered by their lack of access to the decision-making procedures in the biomedical clinic. They may be unfamiliar with the constraints of working under the aegis of a large bureaucracy, where there is constant reference to the rationalization of resources and formal accountability. Most practitioners are more used to working in a market setting, as autonomous individuals or as members of small co-operative groups (Sharma 1995:128ff).

At the same time the worst fears of complementary practitioners do not seem to be realized. The retention of the gate keeping and fund holding role of the GP in integrated primary health care is not incompatible with empowerment of the complementary practitioner provided that this is recognized as something which needs to be worked at. If there is no great motivation to do this on the part of medical staff, it will go by the board in general practice where time is at a premium. Stephen Gordon of the Society of Homoeopaths is right when he warns homoeopaths that while their incorporation into the NHS might have many advantages, they should be aware that GPs may regard their lengthy consultations as less than cost effective (Gordon 1992:8).

Where clinicians and health service managers are under pressure to account for results there is also the danger that they will judge alternative practitioners' performance by standards inappropriate to holistic practice. Whelan points out that the initial experience in the Liverpool Centre for Health was that GPs sent complementary practitioners patients with chronic conditions, who were then seen by the therapists for as long as they continued to show any improvement. This tendency to keep patients on the books, combined with a high demand for initial consultations, meant that there were long waiting lists, just as in other parts of the NHS. While the service was continued beyond its initial six-month trial period, there was considerable pressure on the therapists to achieve a higher turnover of patients. If practitioners cannot work "in their own time" they will not be producing holistic health care, and may not achieve the kind of results that they otherwise could. They then risk being judged unsuccessful by both NHS purchasers and the public. The new focus on "value for money" is

> shifting the emphasis, and with it an entire philosophy, away
> from something that has been potentially truly transformative

to patients. But – it was ever thus – the NHS is not and never has been about empowerment and transformation of patients. As a public service with too few resources for the demand facing it, it cannot afford to be (Whelan 1995:82).

Some doctors who have worked with complementary practitioners are very sensitive to this problem. Two GPs who employed the services of a homoeopath noted that while cost effectiveness was important "the success of the project cannot be judged by the number-crunching approach" and that quality of life for patients was an important aspect of success (Ward 1995:9). At the same time reports by doctors responsible for such projects seldom fail to mention resource savings made through such collaborations, in terms of lower rates of drug prescription, reduction in consultations with the GPs, etc. (e.g. Budd et al. 1990:378, Burns & Lyttelton 1994:203).

Whether or not complementary treatment leads to savings in health care expenditure depends on what kinds of comparisons are made. The Lewisham Health Authority decided in 1997 to stop paying for homoeopathic treatment since, it was argued, the funds spent on referring 500 patients a year to the Royal Homoeopathic Hospital would have allowed 100 patients to have hip replacements (Wise 1997). With the increased emphasis on "evidence" based medicine in many western countries (Visser 1997:12), and the relative paucity of such evidence for many alternative treatments, the problem of the terms of evaluation is not likely to go away. Indeed in a climate where questions about health care "rationing" are starting to be raised it is likely to become even more contentious.

Patient empowerment

Holistic health care is often represented as empowering for patients, who are helped to understand and take responsibility for their own health (Sharma 1994). Some integrated clinics have tried to make this an explicit aim. For example, the Marylebone Centre involved patients as volunteers in the work of the centre, e.g. in helping to produce a practice newsletter, or befriending isolated patients in need of emotional support. This had some success, but was prone to a problem noted in relation to patient participation groups in general, namely that after an initial burst of enthusiasm participation was liable to fall off and become difficult to maintain. Pietroni & Chase note the need to establish a "neutral" ground on which patient/volunteers and doctors meet as equals (Pietroni & Chase 1993).

One way of looking at this would be to say that the only thing that truly empowers people is power, and to invite users to participate in the running of an integrated Centre as volunteers is not the same as offering them a role in the actual management of the Centre, which would be difficult to achieve within the NHS. The Hoxton project (see above), which is only partly funded by the NHS and raises much of its funding from charitable sources, followed a pattern less common in NHS primary health care, although one that is in keeping with official declarations of commitment to patient empowerment and consumer involvement. In the Hoxton Centre patients could become subscribing members of the Centre and active user participation was encouraged. Indeed the management committee consists of user/volunteers with therapists represented but having no voting rights, i.e. a model more familiar in the voluntary sector in Britain than in public health settings. This arrangement was not without problems for the therapists, but they did feel that it was conducive to the increased participation in treatment that most holistic practitioners would regard as important to therapeutic success (Kettle 1993:151). Perhaps it is easier for complementary practitioners to understand and tolerate some cession of control to patients than to medical personnel? However a similar effect seems to have been achieved by a project similar in structure to the Hoxton project (partnership between charitable trust and NHS practice). This project grew out of a collaboration between a GP and an art therapist and was inspired by Steiner's vision of anthroposophical medicine. Patients were often invited to meetings between the therapists and the doctor and came to play a major part in fund raising and the management of the Trust.

> We were hearing countless variations of the theme "I want to take part actively in what is happening to me", just as we were becoming increasingly involved in a project whose continued existence depended on involving others (Logan 1994:155).

Patients began to offer more support to each other, this becoming "the next step in their own healing process".

It may be that projects with a strong community base are better geared to generating patient participation and introducing different kinds of therapies to people who might not otherwise have used them. The Hoxton project was very successful in making complementary therapies accessible to an older age group and other types of patient who would not be seen frequently in private consulting rooms.

The Craigmillar project in Edinburgh was born of the community health movement with its collectivist ethos and was funded by urban aid. Here acupuncture treatment was provided to a dominantly working class population where stress resulting from unemployment, poor housing conditions, etc. were major problems. The treatment was offered at nominal charges and was very popular, and patients reported their positive experiences to their GPs apparently leading to an increase in GP referrals for acupuncture (Ritchie & Ritchie 1991). We might tentatively conclude from these two projects that patients can fairly readily be mobilized to define and manage services in a voluntary sector type organizational setting. However, in these two examples the degree of "integration" achieved is quite low; GPs regularly referred to these projects but they did not work alongside complementary practitioners nor share in management.

The collectivist model of organization favoured in much of the British voluntary sector is only one model of non-statutory collaboration. In the USA many holistic clinics (which would be described as "integrated" in Europe in as much as they group together clinicians of different kinds) are, according to Mattson, the brain children of individuals who have "envisioned one kind of centre and proceeded to organize, staff and manage it", though some are generated by collectives and yet others are church based. Either way, Mattson notes that user involvement in management is rare, though often stated as an aim. There is apparently little uniformity in patterns of management (Mattson 1982: 102–3) though Mattson observes somewhat cryptically that "a few centers have undergone significant changes in the leadership, management or focus as part of their evolution" (Mattson 1982: 104). That tensions between "integrated" clinicians and managers may be highly problematic is more than hinted at in a Finnish study. Antti Hernesniemi, a medical doctor, worked with traditional healers (bonesetters) in the Folk Medicine Centre at Kaustinen. State funds for the project were channelled through a local foundation, and tension arose between the clinicians and the management, dominated by local politicians and business-men, who apparently felt threatened by Hernesniemi's wish to make the Centre a site for scientific research rather than money making (Hernesniemi 1994:135–6).

To summarize, there are many different kinds of organizational context for collaboration. It may take place within the existing state provided biomedical clinic, it may develop from community initia-tives or from the enterprise of private practitioners (though there is little information on this last type). However, in most of the ac-counts available to us it seemed that the doctor was more often (in some sense or other) the senior participant in the collaboration, and that this could not but help colour the direction and type of commu-nication developed both among practitioners and between practi-tioners and patients. This, however, is not to underestimate the novelty and imaginativeness of some of the initiatives nor the possi-bilities they hold for better health care for patients.

Integration as the practice and knowledge of alternative medicine by doctors

An interesting aspect of the vocabulary that has developed around alternative medicine is that when the term "integration" is applied to knowledge it generally refers to the appropriation of alternative medical knowledge by doctors. We have already seen that some therapies have incorporated a great deal of biomedical knowledge into their training curricula. This tends to be treated as unremark-able, no more than what one would expect, whereas the adoption of alternative medical knowledge by doctors is something more special – praiseworthy or controversial according to one's view. This itself is probably a manifestation of the kind of assymetries that are a central problem in this chapter.

If we take integrated medicine to mean medical personnel prac-tising complementary therapies as part of their clinical repertoire then integrated medicine has already been around for a very long time. As we have seen in Chapter 4, there is a high level of interest on the part of doctors in learning to practice complementary techniques. Some have been practising therapies like acupuncture or homoeopathy for years as adjuncts to their biomedical practice.

Complementary practitioners have constantly expressed concern that GPs – on the basis of quite brief training sessions – could be practising complementary medicine to less exacting standards than those required by the emerging alternative professional groups. Indeed this concern was expressed by the BMA in its 1993 report, which stated that

> it was clearly unsatisfactory for medical practitioners who have received little formal training to undertake therapies for which they are not competent. Where there are clear and recognised standards of competence laid down for a therapy, such as osteopathy, the therapist, whether medically qualified or not, should satisfy those criteria (BMA 1993:42).

This issue is beginning to be addressed by the medical educators. David Reilly and his colleagues at Glasgow designed a module in conjunction with the Faculty of Homoeopathy which provided teaching about the general issues involved in the practice of homoeopathy, and a number of "targeted primary care uses" for that therapy. This was offered to qualified doctors as a unit of postgraduate education, and an audit of those who completed the course carried out over two years indicated a high degree of success. Reilly & Taylor suggest that this kind of project can marry "academic enquiry with day to day medical care" in a constructive way. They defend this experiment against anticipated "fears of an erosion of the scientific substance which medicine has fought to create" (Reilly & Taylor 1993:31).

GPs need to know more about the therapies so as to be in a position to advise or refer patients, irrespective of whether they have any intention of practising alternative medicine themselves. Another project initiated at Glasgow was the introduction of discussion groups on complementary medicine as part of the undergraduate medical curriculum. On the basis of the response to this, Reilly and his colleagues designed an undergraduate course to meet the need for greater knowledge about the basis of complementary therapies.

How far should doctors have training in the basic philosophies of complementary medicine (as opposed to being introduced to a few specific techniques which they can safely practice)? Surely only in that way can there be a genuine integration of *knowledge*. Peters urges the need for a postgraduate course which, through comparative study, would "investigate the intellectual and cultural landscape of complementary medicine dispassionately and with appropriate rigour, exploring its interface with conventional clinical science and practice" (Peters 1995:33). Where practice is concerned, he envisages doctors learning from complementary practitioners using an empirical problem-based approach.

But if doctors do need to learn more than just a few superficial techniques, how much more do they need to know and what happens when they come to the point where biomedical and complementary understandings of the health and the body actually conflict? Although Peters and others are right that there may be much common ground, what happens when there is a need to go beyond the boundaries of this common ground?

One answer to this is to attempt to go back one step to the point at which knowledge is produced, to develop research on complementary medicine that is scientifically communicable, yet faithful to the objectives of complementary medicine and relevant to its methods of diagnosis and treatment. While some of those who work on the interface between alternative and orthodox medicine have insisted on the need for randomized clinical trials (RCTS) (Ernst 1994), others have been open to a broader range of forms of enquiry, such that co-operation between alternative and orthodox medicine in the production of knowledge becomes feasible. The well known Munich Model is a project (started in 1989) which aims to integrate research and training at a very high level. It has drawn a network of clinics using alternative medicine into co-operation with the medical academic research community through a system of "Scientific Quality Management", and through the use of a range of research techniques (not just RCTS) (Melchart 1996).

Possibly this kind of initiative is easier to achieve in a country like Germany where certain forms of "natural healing" have long been accepted as an established part of the health care system. But the main prerequisites for the reduplication of such a project are first, alternative medicine clinics with staff who have a desire to participate in and an understanding of scientific research, and secondly, medical researchers who wish to collaborate with them. From that point of view the model does not seem to be unexportable. Another possible model can be found in the Maryland project in the USA. This project has multiple aims, but its activities are contained within the University of Maryland School of Medicine. It aims to integrate different therapies into clinical care in a special chronic pain clinic. It also aims to raise awareness of these possibilities within the medical community through elective undergraduate courses based in the unit, seminars and postgraduate fellowships. It also conducts evaluative research using the project itself as a base for such investigation (Berman & Anderson 1994).

However it is precisely at the level of general theoretical knowledge that the differences between alternative medicine and biomedicine can become more evident. As one doctor points out, describing his own journey "in the twilight zone" between the two, the ideas that unite alternative practitioners and those GPs who have an interest in alternative medicine are usually about stimulating the healing powers of the individual, empathic care, the individual nature of sickness and health, etc. These ideas have currency and authority in the primary care clinic but are little explored or taught in the university based medical academy (Eikard 1996).

Returning to the issue of empowerment, the integration of knowledge will make very little impact on medical dominance if there is no modification whatsoever of institutional arrangements and work organization. Peters (1995) raises the question of career structures. If there is a genuine integration of knowledge and practice, should it not be possible for complementary practitioners to achieve consultant status within the NHS? At the moment such a situation is virtually unthinkable – the public health care system in Britain can incorporate aspects of alternative medicine and can sponsor forms of collaboration within primary and some secondary settings, but non-medically trained practitioners still have no well defined senior roles to aspire to within the NHS, they are always in some sense "outsiders".

To summarize the argument so far, "integration" (in the various senses in which the term is used) has not so far seriously undermined the institutional position of doctors. Where integration means collaboration within the clinic, doctors have an organizational advantage, being more securely anchored in the relevant bureaucratic structures (however these may be organized locally). Where doctors are themselves managed by non-clinicians (as in Britain) this makes little difference to their dominance in the micro-setting of the "integrated" clinic. It is perhaps significant that an influential document on the integration of orthodox and complementary health care pays great attention to issues of patient accessibility and interprofessional communication in the delivery of a "Quality" Integrated Therapy Service, but says nothing about the ways in which complementary therapists might be integrated into the career structures of the public sector or involved in the wider bureaucratic processes of decision-making in the NHS (Foundation for Integrated Health Care 1997). This is not to say that "integration" does not bring benefits to complementary practitioners who, like doctors, can see collaboration as bringing gains to their practice or as solving clinical problems which they currently encounter.

Where we are talking about the integration of knowledge the relationship is still asymmetrical. Accredited training for alternative therapists is more likely to include elements of biomedical knowledge (even if only a smattering of anatomy) than the undergraduate medical curriculum is to contain knowledge about other systems of healing. We have noted some innovative programmes that may indicate future trends, but at the moment medical students normally learn about alternative medicine through elective postgraduate training, not as a part of their basic training. However this situation is changing fast and we see nothing inevitable or unidirectional about these developments.

Medical pluralism and medical dominance: lessons from the post-colonial countries

These issues are only novel where the sociology of the western context is concerned. The literature on medical pluralism in the post-colonial world has much to say about the interaction of different healing systems and the scope for collaboration between their practitioners. In such "pluralistic" systems, is biomedical hegemony a foregone conclusion? If some non-biomedical forms of healing are able to find a secure and recognized role in the overall health care systems of these countries, what are the conditions that are favourable to such a development?

Comparative sociology is always a risky venture since there is the danger of comparing the incomparable, perpetuating simplistic oppositions (west/rest, advanced/backward). However we can use the literature on medical pluralism in the post-colonial world as a comparative resource to suggest instructive possibilities.

In much of the non-western world, biomedicine arrived hand-in-hand with the colonial state, imported to attend to the medical needs of colonial rulers but increasingly offering possibilities for the control and surveillance of colonial populations. The colonial state was, in general, either indifferent or actively hostile to indigenous forms of healing. In many parts of Africa "colonial regimes supported medical missionary efforts to illegalize or severely curtail the practice of 'witchdoctors'" (Green 1988:1127). In South Asia the consolidation of British rule in the mid-nineteenth century undermined the institutions that had supported the survival of Ayurveda and saw a drastic decline in the scope and quality of training for Ayurvedic practitioners. When modern colleges for the training of practitioners were established, it was a more professionalized, eclectic and medically oriented form of Ayurveda that was taught (Leslie 1972).

Political independence did not lead to the breaking of the alliance between biomedicine and the state. However in some Asian countries it did offer an opportunity to re-assess indigenous forms of healing and assign to them positive value as representative of a truly national indigenous cultural form. The best known example is India, where Ayurveda and homoeopathy (not indigenous but virtually naturalized as an Indian form) received state recognition. In Pakistan a degree of state support is provided for training in Unani Tibb. In China, never directly under foreign rule, indigenous forms of medicine, especially acupuncture, are practised in state hospitals (Leslie 1975).

The WHO/UNICEF initiative at Alma Ata in 1978 proclaimed the desirability of using indigenous health practitioners in government supported health programmes, and encouraged use of "traditional" medicine to meet the shortfall in health care, especially for rural populations. This idea met with variable degrees of enthusiasm, but did stimulate a number of initiatives, in the first place involving mainly the training of "traditional birth attendants", and later other indigenous practitioners. More recently, concern with the rapid spread of AIDS has led to a revival of interest in the role that traditional healers could play in health promotion. Some national governments have taken an interest in traditional healers to the extent that they have instituted registers for them, albeit sometimes under pressure from such healers (Last 1990:363–5). In sub-Saharan Africa traditional healers have emerged as vigorous professionalizing groups, eager to seize the "political space" and therapeutic opportunities available to them (Last 1986:11). In Nigeria, for instance, traditional healers can now be registered by the Nigerian Medical and Dental Council (the body which registers biomedical doctors and dentists), the rising demand for their services being in part a result of the increased costs of biomedical care and the declining purchasing power of patients, due to unemployment. As in a number of other countries, pharmaceutical companies are taking an interest in the pharmacopoeia of the traditional herbalist (InterPress Third World News Agency 1998).

However, in the postcolonial countries of the South "integration" has not typically taken the form of projects like the Marylebone clinic in which practitioners enter into close relations of co-operation or referral over individual patients. More commonly it has consisted of attempts on the part of the state to tack "traditional" healers onto a weakly developed state system of biomedicine, providing some elements of primary or obstetric care or health promotion in rural areas where biomedical resources are overstretched.

Do such efforts indicate a loss of confidence in biomedicine, or any radical challenge to its hegemony? One thing that is very clear from this literature is the tendency for non-biomedical healers to absorb such features of biomedical practice as are locally regarded as prestigious or especially efficacious, and which can be transferred to the non-biomedical clinic. Among Ayurvedic physicians in South Asia the prescription of biomedical drugs would seem to be common. Waxler-Morrison, reporting on Sri Lanka, suggests that this is because the

> western institution of medicine has defined the terms of medical practice in the country, including the kind of medicine available and believed to be "good" (Waxler-Morrison 1988:542).

The Sri Lankan government put twice as much funding into the (biomedical) Ministry of Health as into the Ministry for Ayurveda.

An alternative interpretation of this phenomenon is that offered by Nordstrom, who suggests that to define it purely in terms of the dominance of biomedicine is misleading. All that the Ayurvedic practitioners are doing is demonstrating the responsiveness and flexibility of the Ayurvedic tradition, one which encourages individual solutions to individual patients' problems. This is a reasonable position if we agree to treat Ayurveda not as a set of standardized practices based on systematized doctrines, but as a "flexible and multiplex system whose expressions differ among people and change over time" (Nordstrom 1988:488).

"Traditional" systems of healing are therefore traditional only in the sense that they may largely depend for their transmission on informal or unstandardized training, not in the sense that they are unchanging, or inherently conservative.

Indeed it can be argued that the characteristics of a traditional system of healing (or any other body of theory or practice that is transmitted through personal tutelage) are quite the opposite of that ascribed to "tradition" in much western sociology (conservatism, stability); the local guardians of that tradition of knowledge may indeed claim timelessness for their teachings, but "as long as their action follows what Weber calls principles of substantive ethical common sense they are free to innovate" (MacCormack 1986:155). As with the "charismatic" innovators discussed in Chapter 3 it is only with professionalization and the submission to rational legal bureaucracy that this freedom is curbed. Kimani, for instance, comments on the eclectic practice of many Kikuyu healers in Kenya, who have incorporated elements of Islamic and Asian medical practice in areas where they have come in contact with these systems (Kimani 1981:339). Where such borrowing occurs it may be regarded as a product of vigour rather than decadence, and where the borrowing is from biomedicine we do not necessarily have to regard this as evidence of biomedical hegemony. Indeed, there is even a sense in which such borrowing could be taken as a sign of medicine's weakness; neither the medical profession nor governments in such countries have been able to prevent the leakage of biomedical technology, knowledge and practice from the biomedical clinic and academy.

The preparedness of traditional healers to learn from biomedical personnel has been seen as a positive factor in engaging their skills in service of public heath, health promotion, etc., also their potential as "change brokers", mediating between different systems of knowledge (see Green 1988). One of the problems that Green points to, however, is that on the whole traditional healers in Africa may be more interested in access to the prestigious and "high tech" aspects of biomedical knowledge. A study of Swazi healers showed they were interested in learning about the use of X-rays, blood transfusions and injections. They were less enthusiastic about learning oral rehydration techniques, which is what government sponsored workshops offered them (Green 1988:1129). Complementary practitioners in Britain may occupy a holistic "low tech" slot that GPs have abandoned or found it impossible to fulfil, but healers in postcolonial states who can earn a good living in a market created by the shortfall in acute medical care may not be satisfied with this, however well suited their traditional methods are to this kind of care.

Another interpretation is that this kind of eclecticism represents something that we see in another form in Britain. Nichter describes what he calls "masala medicine" – the admixture of Ayurvedic and biomedical practices in the same South Indian clinics (Nichter 1980), very largely in response to perceived demand on the part of patients. The latter may be more concerned with the nature of the medicine prescribed and its appropriateness for the problem in hand than with the nature or status of the system which the practitioner claims to be practising (Nichter 1980:227).

In Britain, it is not uncommon to find complementary practitioners who accumulate qualifications (usually of a fairly low level), adding different therapies to their battery of skills rather than specializing in one. (Unlike the Sri Lankan or South Indian bazaar "doctor", such persons could not hope to add biomedical skills or drugs to their battery of therapeutic resources, there being much tighter control over the availability of drugs and much tighter restriction on, for example, who can administer injections). Accumulation of therapeutic skills is a strategy for maximizing access to patients in a competitive market and the freer the play of patient demand the greater is the impetus to "mixing". Some alternative traditions in the West (chiropractic and naturopathy in North

America, homoeopathy in Britain) have found it difficult to maintain the "purity" of their knowledge under market pressures. In this instance, "integration" (if the admixture of biomedical techniques is to be understood as such) takes place as a product of market forces.

However this does not dispose of medical hegemony. The market is not neutral and pressure from patients on healers to provide biomedical drugs, injections, etc. may reflect biomedicine's increasing status and authority quite as much as a simple continuation of a traditional eclecticism. Myntti's studies of healing in rural Yemen demonstrate that powerful groups in the village profess Islamic orthodoxy yet, in practice, prefer biomedicine to Islamic forms of healing. Indeed they "flaunt" their access to modern medicine, especially their use of expensive imported drugs (Myntti 1988: 519). Morsy reports that even in clinics that purport to provide Islamic medicine in Egypt, what is actually provided is modern biomedicine with a religious label:

> Far from representing an attempt to merge traditional and modern medical approaches ... contemporary Islamic medicine only veils the hegemonic international tradition. Islamic clinics are no different from Islamic banks, Islamic investment companies, and Islamic women's apparel "imported from London" ... within the existing power structure, the placebo effect provided by religious symbolism ... affords the professional "providers" of Islamist health care the opportunity to share power as the state's ideological metamorphosis increasingly lends legitimacy to their efforts (Morsy 1988: 363–4).

Certainly for urban middle class groups, "traditional" medicines may be resorted to for specific illnesses for which they are thought to be effective, but biomedicine is the preferred form for those who can afford it.

Co-operation with indigenous and alternative healers appears to be a strategy that has been more popular with governments and healers than with doctors themselves. In areas like India and China where there are established forms of healing like Traditional Chinese Medicine, Ayurveda or Unani Tibb, some physicians may be highly sympathetic to such systems, probably having had experience of them in their own families. They may recognize them as, if not scientific, then at least based on bodies of established knowledge and lengthy training. Forms of healing that have emerged from folk practice will be less respected and Green has shown that a major obstacle to the co-operation between biomedical and traditional healers in sub-Saharan Africa has been the attitudes of the medical profession (Green 1988:1129). Doctors have felt threatened rather than reassured by the vigorous efforts of "traditional" healers to develop professional organizations with accredited forms of training. Indeed, one can see why this should be so in countries where doctors have the choice between working in a public hospital system that is underfunded and inadequate, or competing in the private market with healers who derive market strength both from the "leakage" of biomedical knowledge and techniques and from a degree of cultural closeness to their patients.

In summary, we see that whereas social scientists researching post-colonial countries have referred to the existence of medical pluralism in the simple sense of "the availability of more than one system of medical therapy", there is far from being parity of esteem among the various systems. The non-biomedical healers may have a good market for their services, adopt innovative and eclectic forms of practice, may even enjoy a degree of recognition by the state, but this is usually within a stratified system of provision where patients' status determines their access to different kinds of healing. There is a tendency for the less prestigious healing groups to imitate the methods of those patronized by elites, i.e. international biomedicine. Some co-operative schemes have been very successful at a local level, but more often due to the willingness of traditional healers to learn whatever biomedical techniques they can manage to appropriate than to any real integration of knowledge or practice. While doctors in the West have seen gains for themselves in adopting and adapting non-biomedical techniques into their own practice, this has happened much less in the non-western world, unless we include the wholesale raiding of the ethnomedical knowledge for new pharmacological possibilities (from which the local hospital or primary care system are likely to benefit very little as yet).

In many postcolonial countries non-biomedical forms of healing were recognized by states in one way or another before the same thing happened in the West. Co-operation between traditional and biomedical healers seems to have been encouraged to meet a general shortfall in the biomedical care provided for the population by·

the state, as well as to meet specific objectives such as AIDS education, education about rehydration techniques, and improvement of obstetric care in remote areas. But where the state has encouraged such co-operation this has not been associated with any decline of the alliance between the medical profession and the state. To this extent we have a comparable situation to that in Britain where non-biomedical healing attracts the interest of those who manage state funded health care in the context of a funding crisis in the NHS and anxiety about the problems of supporting patients with chronic and incurable illness in the community.

However another major factor is popular demand. In the non-western countries we have been discussing, the shortfall in publicly provide health care means that many people, even the very poor, are obliged to buy their health care on the market, a market in which the "traditional" healer probably provides the cheapest deal, even if there is a strong preference for biomedicine in areas like acute illness. "Demand" however can mean political demand as well as "demand" in the market sense. In the non-western world the alliance between the state and the medical profession is not so strong that the state can or would wish to ignore other voices. The desire to be seen to be supporting national indigenous culture and institutions may be an important factor in the recognition of non-biomedical healing groups, especially where this desire can be indulged at no great cost to the state (e.g. the cost of education of traditional healers is still largely a matter for the private sector).

Conclusion

While we must not overestimate the parallels between western and non-western situations, the comparison is nevertheless instructive. On the strength of it we can suggest that integration of biomedical and non-biomedical systems of healing, whether initiated by the state or by healers themselves, does not in itself do away with medical hegemony (as that concept has been understood by social scientists). Integration in the sense of direct collaboration between biomedical and other healers takes place mainly within the framework of existing public health institutions. Here the role of the non-biomedical healer is liable to be one that has been tacked on to the organization of the state run clinic or health promotion scheme. Integrated medicine in the other sense (the admixture of knowledge about different forms of healing) may take place in a variety of contexts – in the western hospital when doctors experiment with the administration of acupuncture to pain clinic patients, or nurses use aromatherapy on the wards. Equally it may take place in the private clinic where health care practitioners of different kinds have an eye to what they perceive as satisfying patients. What knowledge and technology will be borrowed from whom will depend very much on what is accessible, what is deemed "effective" and on what is regarded as attractive to patients. Much of the knowledge transfer will be from biomedicine to other forms of healing, but biomedicine draws in alternative and traditional techniques where these are seen as a useful complement to biomedical practice.

On the other hand, this does not mean that what "integration" has taken place is insignificant, especially when examined from the point of view of patients. We have intended a realistic rather than a pessimistic view. At worst the patients are receiving a form of "masala" medicine. At best they are benefiting from the cross ferti- lization of different traditions of healing and the development of a holistic synthesis.

CHAPTER 7

Conclusion: do we have a new medical pluralism?

Alternative medicine and pluralistic legitimation

At the outset of this book we stated our intention of writing an account of the re-emergence of alternative medicine that went beyond narratives based on conventional medical sociology, an account that would recognize both alternative medicine's relationship to biomedicine but also its situation in a wider cultural and political context. There is no doubt that in "western" countries many forms of alternative medicine are achieving a degree of social legitimacy which they did not have before. In 1977, Cobb described the processes that permitted the "pluralistic legitimation" of chiropractic in America as including; legal sanctions (existence of state licensing, state recognized auto-regulation, etc.); government sanctions (in the form of funding for research, patient reimbursement, training of practitioners, etc.); academic sanctions (acceptance of the therapy as a legitimate subject for teaching and for investigation by researchers); professionalization of the therapists (agreement on a core of theoretical knowledge, service orientation, unified organization, etc.); the support of social movements that question older forms of professional authority; popular demand – i.e. lay users are no longer regarded as or regard themselves as "deviant" (Cobb 1977). The review that we have presented demonstrates that Cobb's analysis of pluralistic legitimation applies to a wide range of alternative medicines today, though not always to the same degree, and in ways which reflect the diversity of institutional arrangements for the delivery and funding of health care in different western countries.

"Legitimacy" in this sense is not conferred solely by biomedicine, even though it is rejection by biomedicine that made therapies "alternative" in the first place; indeed many therapies have faced continuing opposition from many biomedical quarters.

We must, of course, be wary of over generalization. We did not expect at the outset that our account would be unilinear or uniform. The heterogeneity of both alternative medicines and biomedical practice meant that the story we would tell must be multi-stranded. The experiences of alternative medicine vary by therapy, and there may be differences between the perspectives of the official professional representatives of the therapy and the perspectives of the "grassroots" practitioners. The same is very largely true of biomedicine, which emerges as less of a monolithic entity than would appear either from its own self representations or from the way it is represented by some social scientists. We could even say that the boundaries between orthodox biomedical practice and alternative medicine in any given country are not as stable and impermeable as either social scientists or practitioners have made them out to be, and in some countries are clearly in the process of redefinition.

However, it is still true that it is largely biomedical perceptions that have contributed to the driving of a wedge between the better established therapies and others less well regarded by doctors, especially those practised or patronized by minorities or the socially excluded (e.g. Unani Tibb, and some forms of ritual and spiritual healing). This recognition also widens the gap between the practitioners who have a recognized qualification and those who, on the basis of some inspiration and a little knowledge, set up as "healers", often of a non-specific kind. We must remember that the story of alternative medicine is not just the story of the major therapies, though the greater availability of research data on these means that they have had a more prominent place in our account. Overall, the recognition of certain therapies as "legitimate" has meant that the state has been increasingly prepared to legislate where consumers did so before, but also that this recognition has only been granted where therapy groups have undergone a process of "convergence" with biomedicine. Consequently, there may have been a rearticulation of the relationship between the state and biomedicine, but the persuasiveness of the biomedical model in judging other providers remains relatively intact.

The re-emergence of alternative medicine: patients, practitioners, doctors and governments

In the Introduction to this book we stated our aim of telling the story of the re-emergence and increased legitimation of alternative medicines from the point of view of four key agents (or sets of agents) in the field of activity which we called the social relations of health. The material we presented in the chapters that followed shows that alternative medicines have not simply been "inserted" into the field but have benefited from (and no doubt contributed to) some radical shift in existing relations among the other agents.

So far as the users of alternative medicine are concerned, the immediate motivation to use alternative medicine may be pragmatic and related to a specific health problem rather than ideological. Yet we have seen that usage of alternative medicine can be seen as a manifestation of both a more challenging attitude to biomedical authority and of changing perceptions of health care in general. The "patient" is (in relation to alternative medicine, and to a limited extent in relation to biomedicine also) increasingly constructed as a "consumer" who makes choices from what is accessible to him/her which have both rationality and symbolic weight. Possibly patients are "reskilling" themselves in the face of the disempowerment they face from reliance on "abstract systems" and on the professionals that deliver these systems; certainly research shows that users of alternative medicine appreciate the collaborative relationship which some practitioners encourage and find it empowering.

The practitioners of alternative medicine have benefited from consumer preparedness to question professional authority. But to consolidate this advantage they have needed to lay claims to a degree of professional authority themselves. They have sought greater legitimacy in a number of ways – some therapies more as- siduously and more successfully than others. Most have "profes- sionalized" to some degree. Yet, paradoxically, professional status has generally brought a degree of recognition at the expense of acceptance of some biomedical knowledge and standards. Naturally some alternative practitioners have questioned the value of achiev- ing recognition and status at the price of a purely "complementary" role to biomedicine. It remains to be seen whether the smaller and less professionalized therapies will opt for distinctiveness rather

187

than official acceptance, but the trend is to seek greater legitimacy and security.

The biomedical profession has clearly felt threatened by the popularity that alternative medicines enjoy and doctors have had to confront the fact that many of their patients will be using such therapies, often alongside biomedical treatments. Alternative medicine represents one of a number of challenges to biomedical authority, for example those which have issued from the feminist movement, from increased medical litigation, from public anxieties about excessive use of drugs and "high tech" treatments, and so on. At the same time, even if biomedicine has had to abandon its claims to a monopoly of valid and efficacious health care, there is no real threat of a decline in demand for its services – if anything, the reverse. In some countries national medical associations have responded to the challenge of alternative medicines with determined opposition, using every avenue to block legislation which would regularize alternative therapies or employing existing legislation or campaigning tactics to undermine individual practitioners. Yet, while all this has been going on, many doctors, especially those in the primary health care sector, have themselves been interested in alternative medicine, seeing it as helpful for some of the more intractable health problems they encounter in daily practice. Some have learnt to practice alternative therapies themselves, others have sought to collaborate with therapists.

In such circumstances it is difficult for the official representatives of such doctors to maintain an explicitly oppositional stand towards all alternative medicines and at the same time keep their grassroots members with them. Probably more national medical associations will take the tack adopted by the BMA. That is, they will adopt a less confrontational approach while laying claim to the moral high ground as arbiters of good professional practice and to the intellectual high ground as experts in how to determine what is regarded as genuinely efficacious.

Governments, as we have seen, have a limited interest in alternative medicines. Where (as in a number of European countries) existing laws restrict the practice of healing to biomedical doctors, some governments have responded to public pressure to reform the law and have even provided limited funds for research into alternative therapies. In some countries the same effect has been achieved by simply failing to enforce restrictive laws. In Britain, there was no such restrictive legislation, and so a "do nothing" approach succeeded fairly well in balancing the conflicting demands of (on the one hand) public and even parliamentary pressure, and (on the other) the privileged counsel of the medical profession. Various factors, however, have favoured a more positive attitude on the part of governments. One is the issue of health care funding. The demand for (and consequent costs of) health care does not decline with economic development, but rises. It is tempting for those who manage publicly funded health care to see in alternative medicine the possibility of a cheaper form of provision – just as in some postcolonial states traditional healers were regarded as helping to meet a shortfall in health care provision. But more fundamentally, the government in Britain and a number of comparable states has been presiding over a "refiguring of expertise". The modern state requires the expertise of various professions to exercise surveillance and control of populations. Traditionally it has relied heavily on its alliance with biomedicine, and continues to do so. However states have countenanced or even encouraged a modification of the power of highly organized and articulate professional groups working in the public sector, while at the same time being prepared to admit the legitimacy of new forms of expertise which might contribute to what Foucault calls "governmentality'. Alternative medicines, therefore, have benefited from a shift in the social relations of health, specifically relations among biomedicine, government and the citizen-consumer, but they have usually done this at the expense of a certain degree of radicalism.

Alternative medicine and sociological theory

In this book we have concentrated on the British case, yet clearly the resurgence of alternative medicines and their increasing legitimization is an international phenomenon occurring throughout the West. There has been much local variation in terms of which therapies have been most favoured and which routes to legitimation have been most relevant, but there is clear evidence of a very general trend. If the progression of events has not been unilinear then neither has it been totally indeterminate or unpatterned.

Sociological theory in western countries favours broad characterizations and analyses of the direction of change in "advanced",
"developed" or "western" nations. Currently it pitches these characterizations in terms of concepts like "modernity/postmodernity",
"risk society", etc. Can we relate our findings to these wider issues,
without obliterating the national and temporal variations we have
documented? How can we interpret the re-emergence of alternative
medicine in terms of the theoretical pre-occupations of contemporary sociological theory?

First, we can say something about the foundations of authority
and knowledge. One of the problems with medical sociology is that
much recent work takes as a baseline the period around the Second
World War, a period when modernist faith in scientific medicine was
at a high point, a period when in many European countries systems
of public provision based on biomedicine had the long term effect
of boosting the confidence of the medical profession in its quasi
monopolistic and privileged position. Much sociological and anthropological work on health care has tended to describe modern
developments in terms of their contribution to medical dominance,
and tends to take for granted that the privileged political position of
the profession was supported by unquestioning popular faith in the
superiority of modern medicine. In the light of such assumptions,
if biomedicine was obliged to "move over" to accommodate some
forms of alternative medicine, or if the public makes support for
alternative medicine explicit, then this requires specific explanation.
One broad interpretation might be that it indicates a postmodern
decline of the meta-narrative of modern medicine, a pluralization
of societal views about health and how health is achieved. A more
focused interpretation frames the issue more negatively in terms of
demedicalization, the start of a process of deprofessionalizing biomedical doctors' work.

These ideas certainly have some relevance. But, as we have
seen, the problematic which takes medical dominance as the norm is
itself based on a periodization that can be questioned. If we take as
our baseline the very period when alternative medicine was somewhat in decline, then the 1960s can only be seen in terms of a period
of challenge to biomedicine. We have argued that this challenge
undoubtedly existed, but this period can just as easily be seen as re-
establishing a situation "normal" in most modern history and con-

temporary societies, that is, a pluralistic situation in which one form of healing is dominant, but not to the exclusion of all others. While there are numerous studies of the health beliefs of ordinary people from the 1960s and 1970s that certainly suggest that biomedical views of disease and the body were broadly shared by the populace, these surveys do not seem to have asked the questions which would have revealed whether patients thought these views the *only* legitimate ones, or how they regarded other modes of healing. So it is hard to say that belief in the legitimate authority of medical scientific knowledge by lay people in general has given way to a plurality of other views, when we do not know just how unequivocal that faith in biomedical authority was in the first place. From one point of view, while the specific form of medical pluralism we have described is certainly new, in as much as it represents a reconfiguration of powers and knowledges, pluralism in itself is not new, and it may not be postmodern, or even in itself require special explanation if we start with a problematic that does not take the popular foundations of modernism for granted. We would require more evidence of genuinely postmodern attitudes to health care on the part of consumers before concluding that a plurality of modes of healing necessarily constitutes an indication of postmodernity. The literature we reviewed in Chapter 2 suggests that orthodox medicine still has preeminent authority for most people in specific areas of health care, notably the treatment of acute illness or injury.

Nevertheless, from another point of view, there do seem to have been important changes to the basis on which biomedicine can claim authority. Appeals to biomedicine's superior knowledge base or epistemology no longer work as successfully as they did (though this does not prevent biomedical doctors and scientists from making them) not least because of public dissatisfactions with biomedicine itself, which make such strategies now appear transparently self interested. The vociferous public reactions to the first BMA report demonstrate that biomedicine's attempts to promote its own superiority were a failure. Instead the medical profession have had to alter their claims to authority, portraying themselves as the disinterested protector of the consumer. This claim to moral authority has manifested itself in calls for alternative practitioners to prove themselves to be responsible professionals, properly trained and registered. These shifts may have been prompted by the re-emergence of alternative medicine but are perhaps also a consequence of the wider breakdown in trust in scientific knowledge. The failure of medicine like other scientific discourse to offer predictability, certainty and progress and the risks associated with the expansion of scientific knowledge have meant that (if it ever existed) unquestioning faith in the modernist project has been eroded. In turn, the ability of bio-medicine to assert cognitive authority can no longer be assumed. However, the decline of the trust in biomedicine has not been ac-companied by a consequential lack of trust in all practitioners who claim some expertise in health matters. We have seen that (para-doxically) rejection of some parts of biomedicine by the lay public can be associated with a "leap into faith" with alternative medicine. Of course this may be short lived.

We can also make links between the use of alternative medicine and other cultural changes. For example, one feature of some alter-native medicines is that the boundaries between action aimed at restoration of health in time of sickness, action taken to maintain health and vigour in general, and action taken to achieve an aes-thetically and morally appropriate body have become blurred. Many people consult alternative practitioners because they have some troublesome condition which biomedicine has not been able to relieve. However many are beginning to consult for general health maintenance, prevention of sickness, and enhancement of "energy'. Some of the New Age forms of healing lack the specificity of medical treatment and aim at more general adjustment of body and spirit, a sense of moral wellbeing and attunement. We have suggested that the use of alternative medicine is not just about curing disease, but also about the general care of the body and person. This means that biomedical understandings of what counts as health and illness have been broadened. From this point of view (non-medical) alternative healing is not just another form of healing in a pluralistic system, but a subset of a broader family of practices and regimes relating to regulation of the body. These include fitness regimes, body building, plastic surgery and beauty regimes, slim-ming, meditation, yoga, forms of sport, etc. Consequently, holistic healing may be seen as offering to individuals particular ways in which the project of the body may be pursued. Holistic alternative practitioners use the language of health in preference to that of aesthetics, morality or spirituality (though they often use these as well) but they are not narrowly "medical".

This interest in the body may be seen as a matter of personal choice in a world of expanding consumption possibilities, offering scope for playfulness, creativity and jouissance. Indeed critics of alternative medicine have pointed out that it offers even less scope than biomedicine for a social understanding of the causes of illness, and stresses individual rather than collective solutions to health issues. It therefore reinforces rather than transcends the ideological individualism favoured by the "New Right", even if most of its proponents would not see it in this light. But it can also be seen as operating through a set of pressures. Having the "right" kind of body is not a matter of individual choice – there are multiple social and political pressures which prescribe the kind of body that individuals should aspire to, which places the responsibility for achieving these on individuals and even sanctions those who do not achieve the culturally prescribed ideal. From this point of view, holistic regimes do have much in common with medical regimes and can be seen as emanations of what Foucault terms "governmentality". We are under pressure to make sure that we or our infants have all the inoculations governments prescribe, to take note of public health campaigns against excessive smoking, to conform to pressures in the workplace to look fit and slim, etc. There is even the threat of rationing of medical care for those whose diseases seem to arise from excessive eating or smoking, etc. The practices described above, including holistic health regimes, can be seen in this context as an extension of self surveillance.

Another tradition of sociological theorizing would see this self surveillance as clearly related to the interests of capital. According to this strand of theorizing, capitalism in the period of modernity required a system of medical care that ensured that the labour force was free of infectious and debilitating diseases, and medical dominance (the means through which this was achieved) was underwritten by the bourgeois state. From this point of view, the rise of alternative medicine is at first sight anomalous and difficult to explain. If medical power was helping to maintain the capitalist system in this way, how can we understand the apparent weakening of its monopoly? A simple answer is that (as our material in Ch. 6 shows), this dominance is only apparently weakened. Alternative medicine is only admitted for reasons of state economy or in response to public pressure, and then only in a position of subordination to medicine. A more sophisticated revision of this position would suggest that as the nature of the labour force changes, and the requirements which capital has of it, so the form of medical control and surveillance changes. Holistic health care, radical in some respects, is not at all incompatible with bourgeois notions of individual responsibility, and the new stress on personal growth and energy (not just disease) is in tune with the greater stress on self employment, flexibility of work forces, etc. In turn, alternative medicine like biomedicine distracts attention from the social patterning of illness and offers no attempts to improve the social conditions in which people live. Consequently, there is a sense in which alternative medicine, besides liberating and empowering, actually "remedicalizes" many areas of life, and it is not difficult to see that there is a consistency between certain capitalist values and the values inherent in many new health practices.

What is the "new medical pluralism" like and how is it different from the old one?

We have argued that medical pluralism is (in global terms) a normal rather than an exceptional state of affairs, and (in historical terms) is not even a novel phenomenon in western countries – though it has been a marginal issue to western medical sociologists, whose main preoccupation has been with the sources of biomedical dominance. Yet biomedicine never secured a complete monopoly over the provision of health care in western countries. Until around the second quarter of the nineteenth century in Britain (and considerably later in America) there was a flourishing market in many kinds of healing and the modality which was to emerge as modern biomedicine had only a limited measure of advantage over other modalities offered on this market. The fact that many of these have re-emerged and that many new forms have sprung up and flourished might even suggest that we could look at the period of biomedical dominance as a relatively short lived episode.

Yet the form of pluralism that is emerging in the late twentieth

century differs considerably from the "pre-modern" forms of pluralism and for this reason we have referred to it as a "new" medical
pluralism.

First, the diversity to which it refers is highly structured. The
ways in which this structuring is achieved varies locally, but is not
determined entirely by pure market conditions (if by this we mean
considerations of commercial supply and demand). It is a pluralism
in which biomedicine still has a dominant position and still plays a
major part in the process by which different therapies are accorded
different degrees of legitimacy and prestige. There is a marked
difference in status between those therapies that are permitted to
practice within the biomedical clinic, and those for which such a role
is at present unthinkable. (Obviously the way in which this dividing
line between therapists is drawn will vary according to national and
historical conditions). Even the more privileged alternative therapists still practice in the biomedical clinic in a position subordinate
to the medical profession and are invited in as a result of doctors'
approval. Specifically, within the clinic, the practitioner's workload,
contracts and conditions of work are likely to be controlled by
biomedical doctors or their biomedically oriented managers. In as
much as doctors and nurses themselves practice alternative therapies they do so as an adjunct to conventional therapeutic interventions. Outside the biomedical clinic alternative therapists compete
with each other and with the services of biomedical doctors for the
patronage of an increasingly sophisticated and consumerist clien-
tele. They do this from a position of disadvantage since they lack
many of the resources associated with incorporation into the biomedical clinic – though this does not mean that there are not very
good livings to be made.

In Britain, both the acceptability and subordination of alternative therapies to biomedicine are most clearly manifested in the
public sector; most biomedicine is practised in the publicly funded
NHS and most "integration" between alternative and biomedical
health care is taking place at present in the NHS or in other sectors
heavily dependent on public funding. In countries where the funding of health care takes place through the reimbursement of patient
fees through state or state approved insurance schemes rather than
through medicine provided by the state and free at the point of
delivery, a major division lies between those therapies for which

patient fees are recoverable through insurance schemes and those to which this does not apply. In either case the opportunities for different kinds of therapist are very diverse, and user access to some therapies still depends entirely on the patient's purse.

However a combination of factors means that even those therapies that have not been invited to practice in the biomedical clinic and whose practitioners must compete for patients in the private health care market do not escape the scrutiny of the state and do not enjoy the unregulated freedom from accountability which the "quacks" enjoyed in the pre-modern form of pluralism described by Porter and other historians. The new medical pluralism is one that is structured by the emergent configuration of relations among biomedicine, the state and the consumer/citizens.

As we saw in Chapter 6 there are some points of convergence between this "new medical pluralism" and the forms of pluralism found in some postcolonial countries. In the latter, biomedicine has not yet attained the dominance that it achieved in the modern period in "western" countries. In recent decades postcolonial governments have struggled to exercise surveillance of national populations through the agency of the biomedical clinic, in the face of various pressures – not least the epidemic of AIDS and the constraints of "structural adjustment". There has been an increasing tendency to consider the possibilities of incorporating "traditional" healers into the state funded sector, albeit in a strictly subordinate role. The fact that their services are relatively inexpensive (they expect less remuneration than biomedical doctors and their training is not funded from the public purse) favours this incorporation as well as the fact that many of them are well regarded and trusted by substantial sectors of the population. We have a situation comparable to that in Britain and some other western countries where non-biomedical forms of healing present themselves as ways of dealing with both the funding crises of public medicine and the fact that modern economic development brings with it an escalating rather than a shrinking demand for health care. There may be further convergence between the state of affairs in western countries and that in postcolonial countries if the latter "by-pass" the phase of modernist biomedical hegemony experienced by western countries in the twentieth century, though this convergence or globalization of effect will arise from very diverse historical conditions.

In view of all this, the re-emergence of alternative medicine in the West is neither a trivial nor a marginal issue, nor is it likely to be short lived, though we can make no assumptions about its stability or how it will develop in future.

Should we welcome the new medical pluralism?

As we have seen, there has been much public debate about whether alternative medicine should be recognized by the state and about whether and how it should be required to prove its efficacy and professional competence. There has been relatively little debate about the wider issue of the general role of alternative medicines in the kind of system of health care delivery that we want in the next century, how it might be made accessible to more sections of the population and if so which kinds of alternative medicine would be most beneficial.

We could take a libertarian view and propose that people should have access to whatever kind of healing they desire, that it is not up to either the state or to the biomedical profession to legislate on their behalf or interfere with their decisions. If we take this view then efficacy is less of an issue (the user decides what kind of efficacy he or she regards as relevant and makes a consumer choice on this basis). But this supposes that all forms of healing either all cost the same, or are equally accessible to consumers. This of course is not the case, though the pattern of accessibility varies according to the configuration of therapies available in particular locations and the system of health care funding adopted in a particular country.

If we accept that the state should pay for some or all alternative treatment then it is unrealistic to assume that it will not require some degree of accountability from the professionals whose services are paid for from the public purse. Once accountability is demanded, the question arises as to who sets the criteria for public funding or reimbursement, and who decides which therapies or therapists fulfil them. The medical profession has, as we have seen, well developed and influential "machinery" for making such discriminations and has constantly urged the subjection of alternative treatments to the kinds of scientific trial which are used to test the efficacy of new biomedical drugs. Governments have relied

197

heavily on the "insider" advice of the medical profession in the past, though they may do so less in future. In Britain, it is likely that the views of NHS managers will be just as crucial in determining which therapies are regarded as suitable candidates for public funding, and the notion of "cost effectiveness" is as important as "efficacy" in this context. While consumer perceptions are, as we have seen, politically important it is unlikely that user preferences alone would ever decide the issue of which forms of alternative medicine might be provided by the state.

In Britain and in other western countries with a well developed system of publicly provided health care there is increasingly a dual system of provision; some alternative medicine is provided directly or indirectly by the state, while a flourishing and more diverse market sector exists for those who can afford the private clinic. Many of the therapy groups favour this kind of situation, which provides opportunities both for the relatively secure employment of practitioners who can find a foothold within the NHS while leaving plenty of scope for making a livelihood by offering services in the private market. Well established alternative therapists can make a very good living from private clinical practice often combined with money earned from teaching their therapy in colleges or through publications and lecture tours. There are numerous commercial opportunities to be exploited by those who gain a national or international reputation. It is unlikely that the therapy groups will wish to deprive their members of such chances, and many see independence from a biomedically dominated public sector as ensuring freedom to practice the therapy in the form which they regard as pure and authentic.

But as we see in the case of education in Britain, dual systems of provision offer no equity and limited redistribution, and favour the rich over the poor; the poor must be reliant on whatever the state agrees and can "afford" to provide, whereas the rich may choose between what is publicly available and what they can pay for on the market. Dual systems of provision also favour the mobile over the less mobile; we have seen that in Britain the provision of alternative therapies in both public and private sector is, geographically speaking, highly uneven. Alternative medicine could be made more readily available to local working class communities through community based schemes (see Ritchie & Ritchie 1991) or through more accessible forms of health insurance. But the latter option still involves the problem of discriminating among therapies since no insurance company will foot the bill unquestioningly for any therapy that an individual feels like having.

The authors of this book do not assume that all alternative therapies are equally useful or valid; we have our own predilections and experiences here and our research has taught us that alternative therapists cannot be presumed to be either more or less swayed by self interest than biomedical doctors, nor to be either more or less sensitive to ethical and political issues. We do not see biomedical demands for scientific trials of alternative treatments as unreasonable, provided that there is an acceptance that the methodologies that are appropriate for the testing of biomedical drugs may not be at all appropriate for many alternative interventions. And given the paucity of funds available for such trials, can we delay considering questions of acessibility until the efficacy of every last treatment has been defined in biomedical terms and proven to the satisfaction of medical scientists? What we would like to see is more urgency in discussions about the accessibility of alternative therapies and more direct consideration of the users' interests by all the professions concerned. If osteopathy, chiropractic, or acupuncture are any good at all, why are they only patchily available in the NHS? If spiritual healing or crystal therapy or reiki are as good as their proponents wish us to believe, what are the professional groups doing to see that they are available in every town and rural area, and not just in the areas that are close to training colleges or where the local population is wealthiest? If integrated medicine is such a good idea, which professionals are working to see that patients are provided with a comprehensive account of the benefits and risks of both biomedical and alternative treatments for a given condition?

We need a pluralism that will address the broadest patient needs, respectful of the diversity of patient experience and response, not one that has evolved entirely as a compromise answer to problems of public health care funding or as an *ad hoc* resolution of the occupational struggles of different groups of healers (whether biomedical or alternative).

BIBLIOGRAPHY

Abbott, A. 1988. *The system of professions.* Chicago: Chicago University Press.

Alaszewski, A. 1996. Restructuring health and welfare professions in the United Kingdom: the impact of the internal markets on the medical, nursing and social work professions. See Johnson, Larkin, Saks (1996), 55–75.

Alford, R. 1975. *Health care politics.* Chicago: Chicago University Press.

Allsop, J. 1995. Health Policy and the NHS. *Towards 2000.* London: Longman.

Anderson, E. & P. Anderson 1987. General practitioners and alternative medicine. *Journal of the Royal College of Practitioners* **37**, 52–55.

Association of Community Health Councils 1988. *The state of non-conventional medicine – the consumer view.* London: ACHC.

Atkinson, P. 1995. *Medical talk and medical work. The liturgy of the clinic.* London: Sage.

Australian Bureau of Statistics 1992. *1989–1990 National health survey: health related actions Australia.* Canberra: ABS.

Baer, H. 1984(a). A comparative view of a heterodox health system: chiropractic in America and Britain. *Medical Anthropology* **8**, 151–68.

Baer, H. 1984(b). The drive for professionalisation in British osteopathy. *Social Science and Medicine* **19**(7), 717–25.

Baer, H. 1991. The socio-political development of British chiropractic. *Journal of Manipulative and Physiological Therapeutics* **14**(1), 38–45.

Baer, H. 1992. The potential rejuvenation of American naturopathy as a consequence of the holistic health movement. *Medical Anthropology* **13**, 369–83.

Bagenal, F., D. Easton, E. Harris, C. Chilvers, T. McElwain 1990. Survival of patients with breast cancer attending Bristol Cancer Help Centre. *Lancet* **336**, 606–10.

Baggott, R. 1995. *Pressure groups today.* Manchester: Manchester University Press.

Baker, S. 1997. Formation and development of the Aromatherapy Organisations Council. *Complementary Therapies in Nursing and Midwifery,* **3**(3), 77–80.

Bakx, K. 1991. The "eclipse" of folk medicine in western society? *Sociology of Health and Illness* **13**(1), 20–38.

Balint, M. 1957. *The doctor, his patient and the illness.* London: Pitman Medical.

Baran, G., F. Treuherz, C. Marples-Kemble 1993. Trial by media. *Society of Homoeopaths Newsletter* **37**, 14–15.

Baum, M. 1998. What is holism? The views of a well known critic of alternative medicine. *Complementary Therapies in Medicine* **6**(1), 42–4.

Bauman, Z. 1992. *Intimations of postmodernity.* London: Routledge.

Beck, U. 1992. *Risk society: towards a new modernity.* London: Sage.

Bennett, S., B. McPake, A. Mills 1997. *Private health providers in developing countries.* London: Zed Press.

Berliner, J. & J. Salmon 1980. The holistic alternative to scientific medicine: history and analysis. *International Journal of Health Services* **10**(1), 133–47.

Berman, B. & R. Anderson 1994. Improving health care through the evaluation and integration of complementary medicine. *Complementary Therapies in Medicine* **2**(4), 217–19.

Biggs, L. 1992. *No bones about chiropractic.* Unpublished PhD thesis, Department of Behavioural Science University of Toronto.

Blair, P. 1985. The informed patient – burden or ally? *Modern Medicine* November, 26–32.

Bocock, R. 1993. *Consumption.* London: Routledge.

Borchgrevink, C. F. 1994. Alternative medicine in Norway. See Johannessen, Launsø, Olesen, Staugård, (1993), 51–4.

Bordo, S. 1990. Feminism, postmodernism and gender-scepticism. In *Feminism/Postmodernism,* L. Nicholson (ed.), 133–56. London: Routledge.

Borkan, J., J. Neher, O. Anson, B. Smiker 1994. Referrals for alternative therapy. *The Journal of Family Practice* **39**(6), 545–50.

Bouchayer, F. 1991. Alternative medicines: a general approach to the French situation. In *Complementary medicine and the European Community,* G. Lewith & D. Aldridge (eds), 45–60. Saffron Walden: O.W. Daniel.

Bourdieu, P. 1984. *Distinction: a social critique of judgement and taste.* London: Routledge.

Braathen, E. 1996. Communicating the individual body and the body politic. The discourse on disease prevention and health promotion in alternative therapies. See Cant & Sharma (1996), 151–62.

Brenton, M. 1985. *The voluntary sector in British social services.* London: Longman.

British Chiropractic Association 1993. *Chiropractic Report Special Issue* BCA No. 7, 3.

British Medical Association 1986. *Alternative therapy report of the board of science and education.* London: BMA.

British Medical Association 1987. *The BMA guide to living with risk.* London: Penguin.

British Medical Association 1993. *Complementary medicine. New approaches to good practice.* Oxford: Oxford University Press/BMA.

British Medical Journal 1980. (editorial) The flight from science. *British Medical Journal* **6206**, 1–2.

Budd, C., B. Fisher, D. Parrinder, L. Price 1990. A model of cooperation between complementary and allopathic medicine in a primary care setting. *British Journal of General Practice* **40**, 376–78.

Budd, S. & U. Sharma (eds) 1994. *The Healing Bond.* London: Routledge.

Bunton, R. & R. Burrows 1995. Consumption and health in the epidemiological clinic of late modern medicine. In *The sociology of health promotion*, R. Bunton, S. Nettleton, R. Burrows (eds), 206–23. London: Routledge.

Burns, K. & L. Lyttelton 1994. Osteopathy on the NHS: one practice's experience. *Complementary Therapies in Medicine* **2**(4), 200–203.

Bury, M. 1997. *Health and illness in a changing society.* London: Routledge.

Busby, H. 1996. Alternative medicines/alternative knowledges: putting flesh on the bones using traditional Chinese approaches to healing. See Cant & Sharma (1996), 135–51.

Calnan, M. 1987. *Health and illness: the lay perspective.* London: Tavistock.

Calnan, M., S. Cant, J. Gabe 1993. *Going private. Why people pay for their health care.* Buckingham: Open University Press.

Campbell, D. 1994. Letter: Dirty medicine. *International Journal of Alternative and Complementary Medicine* **12**(4), 4.

Cant, S. 1996. From charismatic teaching to professional training. See Cant & Sharma (1996), 44–66.

Cant, S. & M. Calnan 1991. On the margins of the medical marketplace? An exploratory study of alternative practitioners perceptions. *Sociology of Health and Illness* **13**, 34–51.

Cant, S. & U. Sharma 1994. *The professionalisation of complementary medicine.* Project report to ESRC.

Cant, S. & U. Sharma (eds) 1996. *Complementary and alternative medicines. Knowledge in practice.* London: Free Association Books.

Cant, S. & U. Sharma 1996a. The professionalisation of complementary medicine in the UK. *Complementary Therapies in Medicine* **4**(3), 157–62.

Cant, S. & U. Sharma 1996b. The reluctant profession – homoeopathy and the search for legitimacy. *Work Employment and Society* **9**(4), 743–62.

Cant, S. & U. Sharma 1996c. Introduction. See Cant & Sharma (1996), 1–24.

Cant, S. & U. Sharma 1996d. Demarcation and transformation within homoeopathic knowledge. A strategy of professionalisation. *Social Science and Medicine* **42**(4), 579–88.

Cartwright, A. & R. Anderson 1981. *General practice revisited: a second study of patients and their doctors.* London: Tavistock.

Chaitow, L. 1994. Letter *International Journal of Alternative and Complementary Medicine* **12**(6), 4.

Charles, N. & M. Kerr 1988. *Women, food and families.* Manchester: Manchester University Press.

Christie, V.M. 1991. A dialogue between practitioners of alternative (traditional) and modern (western) medicine in Norway. *Social Science and Medicine* **32**(5), 549–52.

Cobb, A.K. 1977. Pluralistic legitimation of an alternative therapy system: the case of chiropractic. *Medical Anthropology* **4**, 1–23.

Coburn, D. 1991. Legitimacy at the expense of narrowing of scope of practice: chiropractic in Canada. *Journal of Manipulative and Physiological Therapeutics* **14**(1), 14–21.

Coburn, D. & L. Biggs 1986. Limits to medical dominance: the case of chiropractic. *Social Science and Medicine* **22**, 1035–46.

Coburn, D., S. Rappolt, I. Bourgeault 1997. Decline vs retention of medical power through restratification: an examination of the Ontario case. *Sociology of Health and Illness* **19**(1), 1–23.

Collins, R. 1979. *The credential society: an historical sociology of education and stratification.* New York: Academic Press.

Cooper, R. & S. Stoflet 1996. Trends in the education and practice of alternative medicine clinicians. *Health Affairs* **15**(3), 226–38.

Copeland Griffiths, M. 1991. *Dynamic chiropractic today.* New York: Thorsons.

Coulehan, J. 1985. Chiropractic and the clinical art. *Social Science and Medicine* **21**(4), 383–90.

Cornwell, J. 1984. *Hard earned lives: accounts of health and illness from East London.* London: Tavistock.

Coulter, I. 1991. Sociological studies of the role of the chiropractors: an exercise in ideological hegemony? *Journal of Manipulative and Physiological Therapeutics* **14**, 51–8.

Coward, R. 1989. *The whole truth.* London: Faber & Faber.

Crawford, R. 1980. Healthism and the medicalization of everyday life. *International Journal of Health Services* **10**(3), 365–88.

Dale, J. 1996. Diversity and unity in acupuncture. Paper presented to the third Social Aspects of Complementary Medicine Seminar, University of Derby, April 1996.

Davison, C., S. Frankel, G. Davey Smith 1992. The limits of popular lifestyle: re-assessing "fatalism" in the popular culture of illness prevention. *Social Science and Medicine* **34**(6), 675–85.

DOH 1989a. *Working for patients.* London: HMSO, Cm 555.

DOH 1989b. *General practice in the NHS: the 1990 contract.* London: DOH.

DOH 1992. *The patients' charter.* London: DOH.

DOH 1991. Stephen Dorrell clarifies the position of alternative and complementary therapies. Press Release, 3 December 1991.

DHSS 1984. *Health care and its costs.* London: DHSS.

Dew, K. 1997. Limits on the utilization of alternative therapies by doctors in New Zealand: a problem of boundary maintenance. *Australian Journal of Social Issues* **32**(2), 181–97.

Donnelly, W.J., J.E. Spykerboer, Y.H. Thong 1985. Are patients who use alternative medicine dissatisfied with orthodox medicine? *Medical Journal Australia* **142**, 539.

Donnelly, D. 1995. Integrating complementary medicine within the NHS: a therapist's view of the Liverpool Centre for Health. *Complementary Therapies in Medicine* **3**(2), 84–7.

Donnison, J. 1977. *Midwives and medical men.* London: Heinemann.

Doyal, L. 1979. *The political economy of health.* London: Pluto Press.

Easthope, G. 1993. The response of orthodox medicine to the challenge of alternative medicine in Australia. *The Australian and New Zealand Journal of Sociology* **29**(3), 289–301.

Eckstein, H. 1960. *Pressure group politics. The case of the BMA.* Standford: Standford University Press.

Eikard, B. 1996. In the twilight zone. A personal report from a medical doctor betwixt and between. See Olesen & Høg (1996), 222–33.

Eisenberg, D., R. Kessler, C. Foster, F. Norlock, M. Calkins, T. Delbanco 1993. Unconventional medicine in the United States. *The New England Journal of Medicine* **328**, 4 Jan 246–52.

Eklöf, M. 1996. "So-called alternative treatment." On the medical profession's views on quackery and alternative medicine in Sweden. See Olesen & Høg (1996), 187–96.

Elder, N. 1997. Use of alternative health care by family practice patients. *Archives of Family Medicine* **6**(2), 181–4.

Elston, M.A. 1991. The politics of professional power; medicine in a changing health service. In *The sociology of the Health Service*, J. Gabe, M. Calnan, M. Bury (eds), 58–89. London: Routledge.

Emanuel, J., B. Warburton, J. Popay, J. Sidall 1996. *A bit of manipulation and a few needles. An evaluation of GP referrals to complementary therapists for musculòskeletal problems.* Public Health Research and Resource Centre: University of Salford.

Emslie, M., M. Campbell, K. Walker 1996. Complementary therapies in a local healthcare setting. Part 1: Is there a real public demand? *Complementary Therapies in Medicine* 4(1), 39–42.

English-Lueck, J.A. 1990. *Health in the new age. A study of California holistic practices.* Albuquerque: University of New Mexico.

Eriksson, C. 1993. Status of research on alternative medicine in Sweden. See Johannessen, Launsø, Olesen, Staugård (1993), 55–63.

Ernst, E. 1994. Complementary medicine: changing attitudes. *Complementary Therapies in Medicine* 2(3), 121–2.

Ernst, E. 1995. Complementary medicine. What physicians think of it: a meta-analysis. *Archives of Internal Medicine.* 155, 2405–8.

European Council for Classical Homoeopathy 1993. *Guidelines for homoeopathic education.* Kenninghall: ECCH.

Featherstone, M. 1991. The body in consumer culture. In *The body, social processes and cultural theory*, M. Featherstone, M. Hepworth, B.S. Turner (eds), 170–96. London: Sage.

Fisher, P. & A. Ward 1994. Complementary medicine in Europe. *British Medical Journal* 309, 107–111.

Foucault, M. 1979. On governmentality. *Ideology and Consciousness* 6, 5–21.

Foundation for Integrated Medicine 1997. *Integrated Healthcare.* London: Foundation for Integrated Healthcare.

Frankenberg, R. 1981. Allopathic medicine, profession and capitalist ideology in India. *Social Science and Medicine* 15A, 115–25.

Freidson, E. 1970. *The profession of medicine.* New York: Dodd, Mead.

Fulder, S. 1988. *The handbook of complementary medicine.* London: Coronet Books.

Fulder, S. 1996. *The handbook of alternative and complementary medicine.* Oxford: Oxford University Press.

Fulder, S. & I. Munroe 1982. *The status of complementary medicine in the United Kingdom.* London: Threshold Foundation.

Furnham, A. & R. Bragrath 1992. A comparison of health beliefs and behaviours of clients of orthodox and complementary medicine. *British Journal of Clinical Psychology* 32, 237–46.

Furnham, A. & J. Forey 1994. The attitudes, behaviours and beliefs of patients if conventional versus complementary medicine. *Journal of Clinical Psychology* **50**, 458–69.

Furnham, A. & B. Kirkcardy 1996. The health beliefs and behaviours of orthodox and complementary medicine clients. *British Journal of Clinical Psychology* **35**, 49–61.

Furnham, A. & C. Smith 1988. Choosing alternative medicine: a comparison of the patients visiting a GP and a homoeopath. *Social Science and Medicine* **26**, 685–7.

Furnham, A., C. Vincent, R. Wood 1995. The health beliefs and behaviours of three groups of complementary medicine and a general practice group of patients. *Journal of Alternative and Complementary Medicine* **1**, 347–59.

Gabe, J., G. Kelleher, G. Williams (eds) 1994a. *Challenging medicine*. London: Routledge.

Gabe, J., D. Kelleher, G. Williams 1994b. Understanding medical dominance in the modern world. See Gabe, Kelleher, Williams (1994a), xi–xxix.

Gaucher-Peslherbe, P. 1986. Chiropractic as a profession in Europe. *Journal of Manipulative and Physiological Therapeutics* **15**(2), 323–30.

Gevitz, N. (ed.) 1988a. *Other healers. Unorthodox medicine in America*. Baltimore: John Hopkins University Press.

Gevitz, N. 1988b. Osteopathic medicine: from deviance to difference. In *Other healers. Unorthodox medicine in America*, N. Gevitz (ed.), 124–56. Baltimore: Johns Hopkins University Press.

Giddens, A. 1990. *The consequences of modernity*. Cambridge: Polity Press.

Giddens, A. 1991. *Modernity and self-identity*. Cambridge: Polity Press.

Gobin, C. 1984. ' Les Maisons Médicales Francophones. Déprofessionalisation de la médicine ou promotion d'un nouveau mode d'intervention illimitée du médical? *Revue de l'Institut de Sociologie (Solvay)* **1–2**, 257–73.

Goldstein, M., D. Jaffe, D. Garell, R. Berke 1985. Holistic doctors. Becoming a non-traditional medical practitioner. *Urban Life* **14**, 313–44.

Goldszmidt, M., C. Levitt, E. Duarte-Franco, J. Kaczorowski 1995. Complementary health care services: a survey of general practitioners' views. *Canadian Medical Association Journal* **153**(1), 29–35.

Good, B. 1994. *Medicine, rationality and experience*. Cambridge: Polity.

Gordon, S. 1992. Homoeopaths in the NHS. *Society of Homoeopaths Newsletter* **35**, 8–9.

Gordon, S. 1993. Vive la difference. *Society of Homoeopaths Newsletter* **38**, 17.

Gordon, S. 1997a. Report. *Society of Homoeopaths Newsletter* **14**.

Gordon, S. 1997b. The regulation of complementary medicine. *Consumer Policy Review* **7**(2), 65–9.

Gordon, S. 1995. Complementary Medicine in Europe. *Eurohealth* **1**(3), 19–21.

Gort, E. & D. Coburn 1988. Naturopathy in Canada: changing relationships to medicine, chiropractic and the state. *Social Science and Medicine* **26**(10), 1061–72.

Grant, E. 1985. *The political economy of corporation.* London: Macmillan.

Greiner, K.A. 1995. The ethics of using alternative therapies in HIV/AIDS. *Aids Patient Care* **10**, 175–81.

Green, E.C. 1988. Can collaborative programs between biomedical and African indigenous health practitioners succeed? *Social Science and Medicine* **27**(11), 1125–30.

Greenwood, E. 1957. Attributes of a profession. *Social Work* **2**, 44–55.

Guardian 1996. Back to our roots *Guardian*, 9 January 1996.

Habermas, J. 1975. *The legitimation crisis.* London: Heinemann.

Hannay, D.R. 1979. *The symptom iceberg: a study of community health.* London: Routledge & Kegan Paul.

Harrison, S., D. Hunter, C. Pollitt 1990. *The dynamics of British health policy.* London: Unwin Hyman.

Haraldsson, E. 1993. Spiritual healing in Iceland. See Johannessen, Launsø, Olesen, Staugård (1993) 46–51.

Hay, C. 1996. *Re-stating social and political change.* Buckingham: Open University Press.

Helman, C. 1992. Complementary medicine in context. *Medical World* **9**, 11–12.

Hernesniemi, A. 1994. Co-work between a medical doctor and a traditional healer. See Johannessen, Launsø, Olesen, Staugård (1993) 126–38.

Herzlich, C. 1973. *Health and illness: a social psychological analysis.* London: Academic Press.

Hewer, W. 1993. The relationship between the alternative practitioner and his patient. *Psychotherapy Psychosomatic* **40**, 172.

Higgins, J. 1988. *The business of medicine. Private health care in Britain.* London: Macmillan.

Himmel, W., M. Schulte, K. Kochen 1993. Complementary medicine: are patients' expectations being met by their general practitioners? *British Journal of General Practice* **43**, 232–5.

HMSO 1987. *Hansard* **489**, col 1379–1416.

HMSO 1993. *Osteopaths Act.* London: HMSO.

HMSO 1994a. *Chiropractors Act.* London: HMSO.

HMSO 1994b. *Hansard* Feb., 1168–1222.

Honigsbaum, F. 1979. *The division in British medicine. A history of the*

208

separation of general practice from hospital care 1911–1968. London: Kegan Page.

Hubble, M. & M. Middleton 1995. A nurse's role in complementary medicine. *Complementary Therapies in Medicine* **3**(3), 173–4.

Huisman, M. 1989. *Chiropractic practice in Britain.* Unpublished MSc thesis, Anglo European College of Chiropractic.

Inglis, B. 1964. *Fringe medicine.* London: Faber.

Inglis, B. 1980. *Natural medicine.* Glasgow: Fontana.

Inglis, B. 1992. Lessons to be learnt from Australia. *International Journal of Alternative and Complementary Medicine* **10**(1), 15–16.

Inglis, B. & R. West 1983. *The alternative health guide.* London: Michael Joseph.

InterPress Third World News Agency 1998. Nigeria-Health: Alternative medicine basks under new recognition. (news item, 12 Feb 1998).

Jain, K. 1995. Swiss embrace complementary medicine. *Nature Medicine* **1**(2), 107.

Jeffery, R. 1997. Allopathic medicine in India; a case of deprofessionalisation? *Social Science and Medicine* **11**, 561–73.

Jewson, N. 1974. Medical knowledge and the patronage system in eighteenth-century England. *Sociology* **VIII**, 369–85.

Jewson, N. 1976. The disappearance of the sick man from medical cosmology, 1770–1870. *Sociology* **10**, 225–44.

Johannessen, H. 1996. Individualised knowledge: reflexologists, biopaths and kinesiologists in Denmark. See Cant & Sharma (1996), 114–32.

Johannessen, H., L. Launsø, S. Olesen, F. Staugård (eds) 1993. *Studies in alternative therapy 1. Contributions from the Nordic countries.* Odense: Odense University Press.

Johnson, T. 1993. Expertise and the State. In *Foucault's new domain*, Gane, M. & T. Johnson (eds) pp 139–53. London: Routledge.

Johnson, T. 1996. Governmentality and the institutionalisation of expertise. See Johnson, Larkin, Saks (1996), 7–25.

Johnson, T., G. Larkin, M. Saks (eds) 1996. *Health professions and the state in Europe.* London: Routledge.

Kelly, M. & D. Field 1994. Comments on the rejection of the biomedical model in sociological discourse. *Medical Sociology News* **19**(2), 34–7.

Kettle, C. 1993. Hoxton health group: a central resource for complementary health care. *Complementary Therapies in Medicine* **1**(3), 148–52.

Kew, J., C. Morris, A. Aihie, R. Fysh, S. Jones, D. Brooks 1993. Arsenic and mercury intoxication due to Indian ethnic remedies. *British Medical Journal* **306**, 506–7.

Kingdom, J. 1990. *The civil service in liberal democracies.* London: Routledge.

Kings Fund 1991. *Report of a working party on osteopathy.* London: King Edward's Hospital Fund for London.

Kirk, A. 1994. The alternative of being alternative. Some contributions to the state registration debate. *Society of Homoeopaths Newsletter.*

Kimani, V.K. 1981. The unsystematic alternative. Towards plural health care among the Kikuya of central Kenya. *Social Science and Medicine* **15b**, 333–40.

Klein, R. 1995. *The new politics of the NHS.* London: Longman.

Kleinman, A.1988. *The illness narratives.* New York: Basic Books.

Kopelman, L. & J. Moskop 1981. The holistic health movement: a survey and critique. *Journal of Medicine and Philosophy* **6**, 209–35.

Koss, J.D. 1980. The therapist spiritualist training project in Puerto Rico: an experiment to relate the traditional healing system to the public health system. *Social Science and Medicine* **14B**, 255–66.

Kotarba, J. 1983. Social control function of holistic health care in bureaucratic settings; the case of space medicine. *Journal of Health and Social Behaviour* **24**, 275–88.

Lagnado, L. 1996. Oxford to unveil its first network of holistic medicine. *Wall Street Journal* October 14th, 2.

Lalli, P. 1983. D'autres médicines; le paradoxe dans le quotidien. *Cahiers Internationaux de Sociologie* **30**(74), 165–8.

Lannoye, M. 1996. *European Report on the status of non-conventional medicine.* Heanor: (Edited version) Natural Medicines Society.

Lannoye, P. 1997. *Report on the status of non-conventional medicine.* European Union: Brussels, 6 March 1997.

Laplantine, F. & P. Rabeyron 1987. *Les médicines parallèles.* Paris: Presses Universitaires de France ("Que sais-je?" series).

Larkin, G. 1983. *Occupational monopoly and modern medicine.* London: Tavistock.

Larkin, G. 1992. Orthodox and osteopathic medicine in the inter-war years. In *Alternative medicine in Britain*, M. Saks (ed.), 112–23. Oxford: Clarendon Press.

Larkin. G. 1996. State control and the health profession in the United Kingdom: Historical perspectives. See Johnson, Larkin, Saks (1996), 45–55.

Last, M. 1986. The professionalisation of African medicine: ambiguities and definitions. Introduction. In *The professionalisation of African medicine*, M. Last & D. Chavanduka (eds), 1–28. Manchester: Manchester University Press.

Last, M. 1990. Professionalisation of indigenous healers. In *Medical anthropology, contemporary theory and method,* T. Johnson & C. Sargent (eds), 349–66. New York: Praeger.

Leslie, C. 1972. The professionalisation of Ayurvedic and Unani medicine. In *Medical men and their work. A sociological reader*, E. Freidson & E. Lorber, 39–54. Chicago: Aldine.

Leslie, C. 1975. Pluralism and integration in the Indian and Chinese medical systems. In *Medicine in Chinese cultures*, E. Alexander, A. Kleinman, P. Kunstadter (eds), Washington DC: John Fogerty International Centre.

Lewith, G. & D. Aldridge. 1991. *Complementary medicine in the European community*. Saffron Walden: C.W Daniel.

Light, D. 1996. Countervailing powers: a framework for professions in transition. See Johnson, Larkin, Saks (1996), 25–45.

Lloyd, P., D. Lupton, D. Wiesner, S. Hasleton 1993. Choosing alternative therapy: an exploratory study of socio-demographic characteristics and motives of patients resident in Sydney. *Australian Journal of Public Health* **17**(2), 135–41.

Lock, M. 1988. A nation at risk: interpretations of school refusal in Japan. In *Biomedicine examined*, M. Lock & D. Gordon (eds), 377–414. Dordrecht: Kluwer.

Logan, J. 1994. The Blackthorn Trust; expanding a national health practice. *Complementary Therapies in Medicine* **2**, 154–7.

Lowenberg, J. & F. Davis 1994. Beyond medicalisation-demedicalisation: the case of holistic health. *Sociology of Health and Illness* **16**(5), 579–99.

Lupton, D. 1995. *The imperative of health*. London: Sage.

MacCormack, C. 1986. The articulation of western and traditional health care. In *The professionalisation of African medicine*, M. Last & G. Chavanduka (eds), 151–64. Manchester: Manchester University Press.

MacDonald, K. 1995. *The sociology of the professions*. London: Sage.

MacEoin, D. 1993. The choice of homoeopathic models. The patients' dilemma. *The Homoeopath* **51**, 108–14.

MacGregor, K. & E. Peay 1996. The choice of alternative therapy for health care. Testing some propositions. *Social Science and Medicine* **43**(9), 1317–27.

MacLennan, A., D. Wilson, A. Taylor 1996. Prevalence and cost of alternative medicine in Australia. *The Lancet* **347**, 569–73.

Mannington, J., J. Moss, N. Josefowitz 1989. Women chiropractors: issues of gender and family. *Journal of Manipulative and Physiological Therapeutics* **12**(6), 434–9.

Marshall, A. 1995. Complementary therapies and conventional practice: exploring the professional boundaries. *British Journal of Therapy and Rehabilitation* **2**(8), 449–52.

Martin, S. 1989. Who's protecting who – and from what? *Journal of Alternative and Complementary Medicine* **7**(8), 21–2.

211

BIBLIOGRAPHY

Mattson, P. 1982. *Holistic health in perspective.* Palo Alto: Mayfield Publishing Company.

McLennan, G. 1995. *Pluralism.* Buckingham: Open University Press.

McMahon, R. 1991. Therapeutic nursing: theory issues and practice. In *Nursing as therapy,* R. McMahon & A. Pearson (eds). London: Chapman & Hall.

Meade, T., S. Dyer, W. Browne, J. Townsend, A. Frank 1990. Low back pain of mechanical origin: randomised comparison of chiropractic and hospital outpatient treatment. *British Medical Journal* **300**(6737), 1431–7.

Melchart, D. 1996. Integration of complementary medicine in research at the University of Munich. See Olesen & Høg (1996), 159–70.

Melrose D. 1982. *Bitter pills. Medicines and the third world poor.* Oxford: Oxfam.

Menges, L. 1994. Regular and alternative medicine; the state of affairs in the Netherlands. *Social Science and Medicine* **39**(6), 871–3.

Mishler, E. 1984. *The discourse of medicine: dialectics of medical interviews.* Norwood, NJ: Ablex Publishing Corporation.

Moore, J., K. Phipps, D. Marcer 1985. Why do people seek treatment by alternative medicine, *British Medical Journal* **290**, 28–9.

Moore, C. 1995. A clash of cultures. *International Journal of Alternative and Complementary Medicine* **13**(7), 24–5.

MORI (Market and Opinion Research International) 1989. *Research on alternative medicine* (conducted for *The Times*).

Morrison, R. 1990. Building bridges. *Holistic Health* **26**, 7.

Morsy, S.A. 1988. Islamic clinics in Egypt: the cultural elaboration of biomedical hegemony. *Medical Anthropology Quarterly* **2**(4), 355–67.

Mumby, K. 1993. Science or flat earthers? The clinical ecologist replies. *British Medical Journal* **307**, 1055–6.

Murray, J. & S. Shepherd 1988. Alternative or additional medicine? A new dilemma for the doctor. *Journal of the Royal College of General Practitioners* **38**, 511–14.

Murray, R. & A. Rubel 1992. Physicians and healers – unwitting partners in health care. *New England Journal of Medicine* **326**(1), 61–4.

Myntti, C. 1988. Hegemony and healing in rural North Yemen. *Social Science and Medicine* **27**(5), 515–20.

National Association of Health Authorities and Trusts 1993. *Complementary therapies in the NHS.* Birmingham: NAHAT.

Navarro, V. 1978. *Class struggle, the state and medicine.* London: Martin Robertson.

Nielsen, J. J. 1993. Integrating metaphors. See Johannessen, Launsø, Olesen, Staugård (1993), 161–73.

Nettleton, S. 1995. *The sociology of health and illness*. Cambridge: Polity Press.

Nicholls, P. 1988. *Homoeopathy and the medical profession*. London: Croom Helm.

Nicholls, P. & J. Luton 1986. *Doctors and complementary medicine. A survey of general practitioners in the potteries*. Occasional Paper No. 2. Department of Sociology, Staffordshire Polytechnic.

Nichter, M. 1980. The layperson's perception of medicine as perspective into the utilization of multiple therapy systems in the Indian context. *Social Science and Medicine* **14B**, 225–33.

Nordstrom, C. 1988. Exploring pluralism – the many faces of Ayurveda. *Social Science and Medicine* **27**(5), 479–89.

Oakley, A. 1984. *The captured womb*. Oxford: Blackwell.

Offe, C. 1984. *The contradictions of the welfare state*. London: Hutchinson.

Olesen, S. & E. Høg (eds) 1996. *Studies in alternative therapy 3. Communication in and about alternatives therapies*. Odense: Odense University Press.

Ooijendijk, W., H. Makenbach, A. Limberger 1981. *What is better?* Netherlands Institute of Preventative Medicine and the Technical Industrial Organisation. London: (trans) Threshold Foundation.

Oths, K. 1994. Communication in a chiropractic clinic: how a D.C. treats his patients. *Culture, Medicine and Psychiatry* **18**, 83–113.

Pahl, J. 1989. *Money and marriage*. London: Macmillan.

Paramore, C. 1997. Use of alternative therapies: estimates from the 1994 Robert Wood Johnson Foundation national access to care survey. *Journal of Pain and Symptom Management* **13**(2), 83–9.

Party Parliamentary Group for Alternative and Complementary Medicine 1993. PGACM Newsletter vol. 1.

Paterson, C. & W. Peacock 1995. Complementary practitioners as part of the primary health care team: evaluation of one model. *British Journal of General Practice* **45**, 255–8.

Pavek, R. 1995. Current status of alternative health practices in the United States. *Contemporary Internal Medicine* **7**(8), 61–71.

Pedersen, P. 1990. The identity of chiropractic practice with special reference to western Europe: a literature review. *European Journal of Chiropractic* **38**, 41–55.

Pedersen, P., P. Kleberg, K. Walker 1993. A pilot study of patients and chiropractors in European practices: socio-demographic characteristics and management procedure. *European Journal of Chiropractic* **41**, 5–19.

Pereira, P. 1993. Medicinas paralelas e pratica social. *Sociologia – Problemas e Praticas* **14**, 159–75.

213

Perkin, M., R. Pearcy, J. Fraser 1994. A comparison of the attitudes shown by general practitioners, hospital doctors and medical students towards alternative medicine. *Journal of the Royal Society of Medicine* **87**, 523–5.

Peters, D. 1995. Perspectives from general practice: skilled doctors or imported complementary practitioners? *Complementary Therapies in Medicine* **3**(1), 32–6.

Peters, D. 1994. Co-operation between doctors and complementary practitioners. See Budd & Sharma (1994), 171–92.

Pickstone, J. 1991. Medicine, society and the state. In *The Cambridge illustrated history of medicine*, Porter, R. (ed) 304–41. Cambridge: Cambridge University Press.

Pickstone, J. 1993. Ways of knowing: towards a historical sociology of science, technology and medicine. *British Journal of the History of Science* **26**, 433–58.

Pietroni, P. 1992. Beyond the boundaries: relationship between general practice and complementary medicine. *British Medical Journal* **305**, 564–6.

Pietroni, P. & H. Chase 1993. Partners or partisans? Patient participation at Marylebone Health Centre. *British Journal of General Practice* **43**, 341–4.

Pill, R. & N. C. H. Stott 1982. Concepts of illness causation and responsibility: some preliminary data from a sample of working class mothers. *Social Science and Medicine* **16**, 43–52.

Pollitt, C. 1993. *Managerialism and the public health service: cuts or cultural change.* Oxford: Blackwell.

Porter, R. 1985. Laymen, doctors and medical knowledge in the eighteenth century: the evidence of the gentleman's magazine. In *Patients and practitioners: lay perceptions of medicine in pre-industrial society*, R. Porter (ed.), 283–314. Cambridge: Cambridge University Press.

Porter, R. 1989. *Health for sale: quackery in England 1650–1850.* Manchester: Manchester University Press.

Pretorius, E. 1993. Alternative medicine in South Africa. *South African Journal of Sociology* **24**(1), 13–17.

Primarolo, D. 1992. *Complementary therapies with the NHS.* London: Labour Party.

Ramsey, M. 1996. Alternative medicine in modern France. Paper delivered at Wellcome Institute for the History of Medicine Symposium on Alternative Medicine in Modern Europe, London, October 1996.

Ranade. W. 1994. *A future for the NHS. Health care in the 1990s.* Longman: London.

Rankin-Box, D. 1993. Innovation in practice: complementary therapies in nursing. *Complementary Therapies in Medicine* **1**(1), 30–33.

Ray, A. B. 1993. Alternative allergy and the General Medical Council. *British Medical Journal* **306**, 122–4.

Research Council for Complementary Medicine 1989. New Sponsor for the Newsletter, RCCM *Newsletter* No. 16, 2.

Research Council for Complementary Medicine 1992. *Complementary therapies. A survey of* MPS. London: Research Council for Complementary Medicine.

Research Surveys of Great Britain 1984. *Omnibus survey on alternative medicine*. London: RSGB.

Reason, P. 1991. Power and conflict in multidisciplinary collaboration. *Complementary Medical Research* **5**(3), 144–50.

Reason, P. 1995. Complementary practice at Phoenix Surgery: first steps in co-operative enquiry. *Complementary Therapies in Medicine* **3**(1), 37–41.

Reilly, D., M. Taylor 1983. Young doctors' views on alternative medicine. *British Medical Journal* **287**, 337–9.

Reilly, D. & M. Taylor 1993. Developing integrated medicine. Report of the RCCM Fellowship, Glasgow University 1987–1990. *Complementary Therapies in Medicine* **1**(1), 3–41.

Reilly, D. T., M. A. Taylor, C. McSharry, T. Aitkinson 1986. Is homoeopathy a placebo response? Controlled trial of homoeopathic potency, with pollen in hayfever as a model. *Lancet* **287**, 337–9.

Richardson, J. 1996. Non-conventional therapy in the NHS: can it work? *International Journal of Alternative and Complementary Medicine* **14**(7), 20–21.

Ritchie, R. & D. Ritchie 1991. The Craigmillar health project: helping people to define their own health needs. *Complementary Medical Research* **5**(3), 160–4.

Rodriguez, J. 1996. The politics of the Spanish medical profession: democratisation and the construction of the national health system. See Johnson, Larkin, Saks (1996), 141–62.

Rustin, D. 1989. The politics of post-fordism: or the trouble with "new times". *New Left Review* **21**, 55–77.

Ryan, S. 1994. State registration to state regulation – the Thin Line. *Society of Homoeopaths Newsletter* **42**, 10.

Saks, M. 1995. *Professions and the public interest. Medical power, altruism and alternative medicine.* London: Routledge.

Saks, M. 1996. The changing response of the medical profession to alternative medicine in Britain. A case of altruism of self-interest? See Johnson, Larkin, Saks (1996) 103–16.

Sale, D. 1995. *Overview of legislative developments concerning alternative health care in the United States.* Michigan: Fretzer Institute.

Salmon, J., H. Warren, H. Berliner 1980. Health policy implications of the holistic health movement. *Journal of Health Politics, Policy and Law* **5**(3), 535–53.

Samson, C. 1995. The fracturing of medical dominance in British psychiatry. *Sociology of Health and Illness* **17**(2), 245–69.

Saunders, P. 1988. The sociology of consumption: a new research agenda. In *The sociology of consumption: an anthology*, P. Otnes (ed.) New Jersey: Humanities Press.

Savage, M., J. Barlow, P. Dickins, T. Fielding. 1992. *Property, bureaucracy and culture: middle class formation in contemporary Britain.* London: Routledge.

Sawyer, C. & J. Ramlow 1984. Attitudes of chiropractic patients: a preliminary survey of patients receiving care in a chiropractic teaching clinic. *Journal of Manipulative and Physiological Therapeutics* **7**(13), 157–63.

Sayyid, B. 1997. *A fundamental fear: Eurocentrism and the emergence of Islam.* London: Zed Press.

Scott, A. 1998. Homoeopathy as a feminist form of medicine. *Sociology of Health and Illness* **20**(2), 191–215.

Sellerberg, A. 1991. Hawks in Swedish medical care: a study of alternative therapists. *Research in the Sociology of Health Care* **9**, 191–205.

Sermeus, G. 1987. *Alternative medicine in Europe. A quantitative comparison of the use and knowledge of alternative medicine and patient profiles in nine european countries.* Brussels: Belgian Consumers' Association.

Sharma, U. 1992. *Complementary medicine today. Practitioners and patients.* London: Routledge.

Sharma, U. 1993. Contextualising alternative medicine. The exotic, the marginal and the perfectly mundane. *Anthropology Today* **9**(3), 13–18.

Sharma, U. 1994. The equation of responsibility: complementary practitioners and their patients. See Budd & Sharma (1994), 82–103.

Sharma, U. 1995. *Complementary medicine today. Practitioners and patients* (revd edn). London: Routledge.

Sharma, U. 1996a. Using complementary therapies: a challenge to modern medicine. In Modern medicine: lay perspectives and experiences, S. J. Williams and M. Calnan (eds).

Sharma, U. 1996b. Situating homoeopathic knowledge: Legitimation and the cultural landscape. See Cant & Sharma (1996), 165–85.

Shilling, C. 1993. *The body and social theory.* London: Sage.

Singer, M. & H. Baer 1995. *Critical medical anthropology.* Amityville, NY: Baywood Publishing.

Skrabanek, S, 1984. Acupuncture and the age of unreason. *Lancet* **1**, 1169–71.

BIBLIOGRAPHY

Smith, T. 1983. Alternative medicine (editorial). *British Medical Journal* **287**, (6388) 307.

Society of Homoeopaths 1997. Editorial, *Society of Homoeopaths Newsletter*, 1.

Society of Homoeopaths 1997. *Code of Ethics*. Northampton: Society of Homoeopaths.

Stacey, M. 1988. *The sociology of health and healing*. London: Unwin Hyman.

Stacey, M. 1994. Collective therapeutic responsibility. Lessons from the GMC. See Budd & Sharma (1994), 107–34.

Stacey, M. 1976. The health service consumer: A sociological misconception. In *The sociology of the NHS*, M. Stacey (ed.), 194–200. Keele: Sociological Review Monograph 22.

Stacey, M. 1988. Research in complementary medicine: a comment. *Caduceus* **5**, 21–3.

Stacey, M. 1991. The potential of social science for complementary medicine: some introductory reflections. *Complementary Medical Research* **5**(3), 183–6.

Stacey, M. 1990/1. A note on the scientific merit of the research. *Caduceus* **12**, 5–6.

Staugård, F. 1993. The role of traditional and complementary therapy in primary health care. See Johannessen, Launsø, Olesen, Staugård (1993), 84–93.

Steffen, V. 1993. Spirits and spirituality: Alcoholics Anonymous and the Minnesota model in Denmark. See Johannessen, Launsø, Olesen, Staugård (1993), 77–84.

Strathern, A. 1989. Health care and medical pluralism: cases from Mount Hagen. In *A continuing trial of treatment*, S. Frankel & G. Lewis (eds), 141–54. Dordrecht: Kluwer.

Suvorinova, L. 1990. If Rasputin had been a Russian TV star. *Journal of Alternative and Complementary Medicine* **8**(5), 15–16.

Taylor, C. R. 1984. Alternative medicine and the medical encounter in Britain and the United States. In *Alternative medicines. Popular and policy perspectives,* Warren Salmon, J (ed.), 191–228. London: Tavistock.

Thomas, K., J. Carr, L. Westlake, B. Williams 1991. Use of non-conventional and orthodox health care in Great Britain. *British Medical Journal* **302**, 207–10.

Thomas, K., K. Fall, G. Parry, J. Nicholl 1995. *National survey of access to complementary health care via general practice*. Sheffield University: Medical Care Research Unit.

Thomas, R. 1989. Editorial comment. *Journal of Alternative and Complementary Medicine* **7**(6), 5.

BIBLIOGRAPHY

Thomas, R. & M. Bishop 1990. Bristol to change after shock report. *Journal of Alternative and Complementary Medicine* **8**(11), 10–11.

Thomas, R. 1990a. "Sorry, but we'd rather not know". Interview with Stephen Dorrell, Junior Health Minister. *Journal of Alternative and Complementary Medicine* **8**(12), 14–19.

Thomas, R. 1990b. "Just let me say" (Editorial). *Journal of Alternative and Complementray Medicine* **8**(10), 5.

Traverso, D. 1993. La pratique médicale alternative. L'expérience de l'homéopathie et de l'acupuncture. *Sociologie du Travail* **35**(2), 181–98.

Treuherz, G. 1990. International outcry follows banning of homoeopathy in North Carolina. *Journal of Alternative and Complementary Medicine* **8**, 19.

Trevelyan, J. 1996. A true complement? *Nursing Times* **92**(5), 42–3.

Van Teijlingen, E. & L. Van der Hulst 1996. Midwifery in the Netherlands: more than a semi profession? See Johnson, Larkin, Saks (1996), 178–87.

Vaskilampi, T. 1993. Alternative medicine in Finland – an overview on the role of alternative medicine and its research in Finland. See Johannessen, Launsø, Olesen, Staugård (1993), 40–46.

Verhoef, M. J. 1996. Complementary medicine and the general practitioner: Challenges for health policy. *Complementary Medicine International* **3**(3), 13–17.

Vincent, C. & A. Furnham 1996. Why do people turn to complementary medicine? An empirical study. *British Journal of Clinical Psychology* **35**, 37–48.

Visser, J. 1991. Communication between general practitioners and alternative practitioners. *Complementary Medical Research* **5**(3), 172–7.

Visser, J. 1997. Cause for pause. *Journal of Alternative and Complementary Medicine* **15**(6), 9–14.

Vithoulkas, G. 1980. *The science of homoeopathy.* New Delhi: B. Jain.

Waddington, I. 1984. *The medical profession in industrial revolution.* Ireland: Gill & MacMillan.

Walker, M. 1993. *Dirty medicine: science, big business and the assault on natural health care.* London: Slingshot Publications.

Wall, A. 1996. *Health care systems in liberal democracies.* London: Routledge.

Ward, A. 1995. *Report on a homoeopathy project in an NHS practice.* Northampton: Society of Homoeopaths.

Wardwell, W. 1992. *History and evolution of a new profession.* St Louis: Moseby Year Book.

Wardwell, W. 1994. Alternative medicine in the United States. *Social Science and Medicine* **38**(8), 1061–8.

Watson, J. 1995. Nursing's caring-healing paradigm as exemplar for alternative medicine? *Alternative Therapies* **1**(3), 26–42.

Waxler-Morrison, N. 1988. Plural medicine in Sri Lanka: do Ayurvedic and western medical practices differ? *Social Science and Medicine* **27**(5), 531–44.

Weber, M. 1968. *Economy and society.* New York: Bedminster Press.

West, P. 1976. The physician and the management of childhood epilepsy. In *Studies in Everyday Medical Life*, M. Wadsworth & D. Robinson (eds), 13–31. Oxford: Martin Robertson.

West Yorkshire Health Authority 1994. *Complementary Therapies and the NHS. Added Value.* (Conference Report).

Wharton, R. & G. Lewith, 1986. Complementary medicine and the general practitioner. *British Medical Journal* **292**, 1498–500.

Whelan, J. 1995. Complementary therapies and the changing NHS: a Development Officer's view. *Complementary Therapies in Medicine* **3**(2), 79–83.

Whitelegg, M. 1996. The Comfrey controversy. See Cant & Sharma (1996), 66–87.

WHICH? 1986. Magic or medicine? *WHICH?* 443–7.

WHICH? 1992. Alternative medicine on trial. *WHICH?* 102–5.

WHICH? 1995. Healthy choice. *WHICH?* 8–11.

Wiles, R. & J. Higgins 1996. Doctor-patient relationships in the private sector: Patients' perceptions. *Sociology of Health and Illness* **18**(3), 341–56.

Williams, G. 1984. The genesis of chronic illness: narrative reconstruction. *Sociology of Health and Illness* **6**, 175–200.

Williams, G. & J. Popay 1994. Lay knowledge and the privileging of experience. See Gabe, Kelleher, Williams (1994), 118–40.

Williams, S. 1989. Holistic nursing. In *Examining holistic medicine,* D. Stalker & C. Glymour (eds), 49–66. Buffalo: Prometheus Books.

Williams, S. & M. Calnan 1996. *Modern medicine: lay perspectives and experiences.* London: UCL Press.

Willis, E. 1989. *Medical dominance.* Sydney: Allen & Unwin.

Wise, J. 1997. Health authority stops buying homoeopathy. *British Medical Journal* **314**, 1574.

Witz, A. 1992. *Professions and patriarchy.* London: Routledge.

Witz, A. 1994. The challenge of nursing. See Gabe, Kelleher, Williams (1996), 23–45.

Wolff, E. 1992. Le rôle du movement des non-médicins dans le développement de l'homéopathie en Allemagne. In *Patients at Militants de l'Homéopathie (1800–1940)*, O. Faure (ed.), 197–230. Lyon: Presses Universitaires de Lyon.

219

BIBLIOGRAPHY

Wolpe, P. 1990. The holistic heresy: strategies of ideological challenge in the medical profession. *Social Science and Medicine* **31**(8), 913–23.

Wright, P. 1988. The social construction of infant care as a medical problem in England in the years around 1900. In *Biomedicine examined*, M. Lock & D. Gordon (eds), 299–330. Dordrecht: Kluwer.

Yu, M., P. Vandiver, J. Farmer 1994. Alternative medicine and patient satisfaction. A consumer survey of acupuncture, chiropractic and homoeopathic health care services. *International Journal of Alternative and Complementary Medicine* **12**(9), 25–8.

Zborowski, M. 1952. Cultural components in response to pain. *Journal of Social Issues* **8**, 16–30.

Zola, I. K. 1973. Pathways to the doctor: from person to patient. *Social Science and Medicine* **7**, 677–89.

INDEX